"Dr. Kornmehl has done a remarkable service to the civilized world in her book, *The Best News about Radiation Therapy: How to Cope and Survive*. She has made available a vast amount of knowledge in plain, easily understood English to satisfy not only the most curious, most inquisitive, but also the most worried patient. The book, in my opinion, is long overdue."
– The Amazing Kreskin

THE BEST NEWS ABOUT RADIATION THERAPY

HOW TO COPE AND SURVIVE

CAROL L. KORNMEHL, M.D., F.A.C.R.O.

ACADEMIC RADIATION ONCOLOGY PRESS
HOWELL, NEW JERSEY

Published by:
    Academic Radiation Oncology Press
    103 Candlewood Commons
    Howell, NJ 07731
    Phone: 732-364-1323
    Fax: 732-364-6950
    E-mail: Info@RTSupportDoc.com
    URL: www.rtsupportdoc.com

ISBN: 0-9721896-0-2
Library of Congress Control Number: 2003101277

Printed in the United States of America

Book design by Janice Phelps

Photos have been used with the permission of:
    Varian Medical Systems, Palo Alto, CA
    MED-TEC, Inc., Orange City, IA
    Philips Medical Systems, Bothell, WA
    Siemens Medical Solutions USA, Iselin, NJ
    Sage Products, Inc., Cary, IL
    Matthew Thomas, Farmingdale, NJ
    Huestis Medical, Bristol, RI
    Nucletron Corporation, Columbia, MD
    Radionics, Burlington, MA

"Without a Song..." Used with permission from EPE.
Cartoon on page X printed with permission from *Not Now. . . I'm Having a No
Hair Day!* by Christine K. Clifford, CSP (University of Minnesota Press, 1996).

This book is dedicated to all patients
— and their families —
who are coping with cancer.

DISCLAIMER

This book is not intended to serve as a substitute for a physician, nor does the author intend to give medical advice contrary to that of an attending physician.

DISCLOSURE

The author has received no grants and has no consulting agreements, speakers bureau membership, stock ownership, or any other special relationships with proprietary entities that have a direct relationship to the subject matter. The author also has no unlabeled or investigational uses of therapeutic products that are discussed in this book.

CONTENTS

Contents

"Adversity strengthens you emotionally and spiritually. It makes you grow into a better person."
– Heather Kornmehl

PREFACE:

WHY I BECAME A RADIATION ONCOLOGIST

My father was a pharmacist, a very strong inspiration to me. From the time I was six years old I knew the names of almost all the antibiotics and antihistamines on the market.

The summer before I started high school, I knew I wanted to become a physician. I was very focused and committed to reaching this highly competitive goal, which I believe helped me succeed academically and socially. My dream came true in my senior year of college, when I received my acceptance letter to the College of Medicine of the State University of New York at Downstate Medical Center.

In medical school, everything seemed to go my way until the middle of my third year. My father was diagnosed with acute leukemia. He spent 60 days in the hospital, and his suffering tore at my heart. In addition to continuing to strive to succeed in school, which in itself was a full-time job, I was my father's advocate because of my medical training. Eventually my father's illness went into remission and he was discharged from the hospital.

Although I was born and raised with the values of caring and compassion, this experience heightened my sensitivity. I realized shortly thereafter that my calling was to be a leader in the war against cancer. Hence, I chose to become a radiation oncologist.

My father did very well for several years, and I was grateful that he lived to see and enjoy many wonderful milestones in my life. I graduated from medical school in 1984, and earned a highly competitive residency in radiation oncology. At my wedding in 1985, both he and my mother walked me down the aisle. He saw me excel at my residency training and pass my written boards.

Unfortunately, my father's disease recurred in 1987 while I was preparing for my written board examination. In retrospect, I don't know how I got through them. Just three weeks after I sat for the exam he needed to be admitted to the hospital. Again, his stay was exactly 60 days, ten days of which were spent in the Intensive Care Unit. Sadly, he lost his valiant battle with cancer on January 10, 1988.

I channeled my grief constructively by concentrating on passing my oral boards examination, which occurred shortly after his death. I reasoned that giving my utmost to this endeavor was a way of paying homage to my father's memory. When I completed my residency that June, my chairman revealed to me that I was the top resident and had scored among the top in the nation on my oral boards.

Words cannot describe how I regretted my father's not being able to witness my latest successes. I also regret that he never got to see and hold any of my three terrific children. As a spiritual person, however, I believe he is aware of these events.

By being who and what I am, I feel I am perpetuating the values that were important to my father. I am proud to say that my passion for radiation oncology has been an inspiration to three other physicians, who changed their intended specialties to similarly become radiation oncologists.

ACKNOWLEDGMENTS

I would like to express my gratitude to my husband, Marvin A. Kornmehl, D.D.S., who inspired me to write this book. His professionalism, wit, and integrity render him a role model for all clinicians.

To my children, Heather, Tyler, and Chelsea, for their unconditional love, patience, and understanding while I was preparing this manuscript — thank you.

My parents, Harold and Bella Lipshitz, nurtured my dream to become a physician and taught me that caring and compassion are just as important as intelligence and honesty. Thank you for such a foundation.

Rosina Rivenberg provided tireless transcription of this manuscript. Thank you for the excellent work.

Also, I am grateful to my entire staff for the personal and meticulous care provided to my patients.

Ellen Kornmehl, M.D., my sister-in-law, provided editorial assistance, which was greatly appreciated. I am honored that she followed in my footsteps and became an outstanding radiation oncologist.

My close friends, Eric Hoffman and Joanne Sinsky, also gave generously of their time with editorial assistance.

Needless to say, I am thankful to the thousands of patients — and the physicians who referred them to me — who have entrusted me with their lives.

– Carol L. Kornmehl, M.D., F.A.C.R.O.

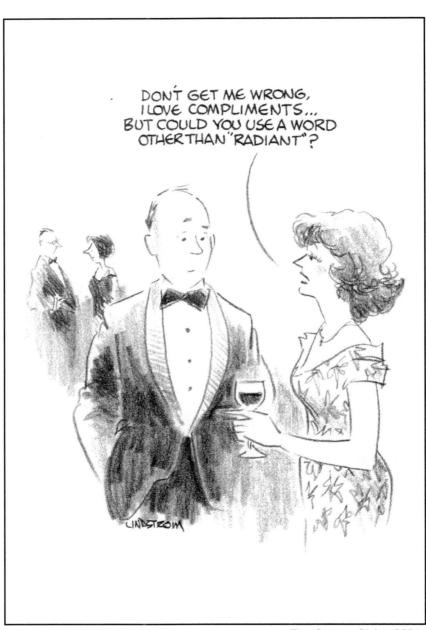

"Knowledge is power."
– Francis Bacon

INTRODUCTION

How did you feel when you were told you needed radiation therapy? Tony was surprised. Kate was shocked. Josephine felt disappointed, intimidated, and worried. Dominic was confused. Genevieve felt devastated and angry. Peggy was neutral and, in fact, was relieved. Richard felt sad.

These are all normal emotions. The good news is that what prospective radiation therapy patients think of as a traumatic experience usually turns out to be less burdensome than anticipated. Misinformation about radiation therapy abounds, but perhaps this book will help to debunk those myths.

I have been practicing radiation oncology since 1988. I am the medical director of a very busy private practice in which I devote virtually all of my time to direct patient care. I love what I do.

Over the years, I hear the same questions whenever I meet a new patient. Among the most common are: "Will I get burned?" "Will I get sick?" "Will I lose my hair?" These might be among your questions, as well.

Radiation oncology is perhaps a patient's least understood area of medicine. Fear and a lack of knowledge make patients feel so vulnerable. Whether you are the patient needing radiation treatment or you have a loved one who needs it, learning what radiation therapy entails will help you begin on a positive note. This book gives you the information you need to become a proactive partner with your treatment team. For those embarking on a course of radiation, I hope the information in this book reduces your anxiety as it guides you through the process.

Note:
*Terms printed in **bold** face are defined in the Glossary*
at the end of this book.

"Start by doing what's necessary,
then do what's possible,
and suddenly you are doing the impossible."
– Saint Francis of Assisi

CHAPTER 1:

WHY DO YOU NEED RADIATION THERAPY?

R adiation therapy is used to treat cancers and some **benign** diseases. Most of the time, the patients I see are referred to me by another doctor. As a **radiation oncologist**, I use my expertise to decide if radiation therapy is appropriate.

A radiation oncologist is a physician who has been specially trained in the principles and practice of oncology, using radiation as a tool to attack cancer. We work together with **medical oncologists**, who are trained at using chemotherapy to fight cancers, and **surgical oncologists**, who perform operations to remove cancers. We work as a team to provide comprehensive, **multimodality therapy.**

When I prescribe radiation therapy, I do so because it is indicated for the cure, the **palliation** (easing of symptoms), or the **local control** of a malignant disease. Many cancers are curable with radiation therapy alone, or with radiation therapy in conjunction with surgery and/or chemotherapy.

Hodgkin's disease is a type of cancer that can be cured with only chemotherapy, radiation therapy, or with chemotherapy and radiation therapy combined. Any therapy used as the only treatment is called the **primary therapy** or **definitive therapy.**

WHY DO YOU NEED RADIATION THERAPY?

Lauren was 12 years old when she was treated with primary radiation therapy for early stage Hodgkin's disease. Today, she is a successful wife, mother, and physician.

Stephen was 27 years old when he was treated with combination chemotherapy and radiation therapy for advanced Hodgkin's disease. His tumors shrunk and disappeared before our eyes.

Sometimes when a tumor has been surgically removed or eliminated with chemotherapy, the referring physician might be concerned about tumor **recurrence**. A tumor might recur if some cancerous cells have been left behind. A cancer's regrowth in the immediate vicinity of the original tumor is known as a local recurrence. A cancer's regrowth in **lymph nodes** is known as a regional recurrence.

Cells can multiply and grow back as aggressive tumors under certain circumstances: if radiation therapy is not administered to the local area; or if lymph nodes that harbor **microscopic disease** are not **irradiated** (treated with radiation).

When radiation therapy is prescribed in the setting where no cancer is detectable but a substantial risk of local and/or regional recurrence exists, the treatment is termed **adjuvant therapy**. A common scenario for adjuvant therapy is the use of radiation therapy after a breast tumor has been removed and the breast has been preserved. Roseanne, a 63-year-old librarian, opted for breast-conserving surgery. She underwent a **lumpectomy** to remove her non-invasive breast cancer, and once her surgical wound healed, she began adjuvant radiation therapy.

Adjuvant therapy occurring in conjunction with surgery is also termed **post-operative radiation therapy**. Post-operative radiation therapy is often necessary if there is not an adequate amount of normal **tissue** (a group of similar cells and the substance between them) at the **margins**, the edges of the tumor.

Radiation therapy may be used before surgery to shrink a tumor and to make the tumor more amenable to removal. Such treatment is called **pre-operative** or **neo-adjuvant radiation therapy**. Pre-operative radiation therapy is often used for head and neck cancers and rectal cancers, and many times it is combined with chemotherapy.

Diane, a 74-year-old crafter of Victorian dolls, is currently receiving chemotherapy in conjunction with pre-operative radiation therapy for rectal cancer. By doing so, Diane is increasing the likelihood that she will not require a colostomy when she undergoes surgery one month after radiation therapy has been completed.

Palliation is a term used to describe therapy intended not to cure disease but to help control its symptoms. Radiation therapy can be used to control and eradicate the symptoms of bleeding cancers or obstructing or painful malignant primary or metastatic cancers. For example, a painful bone **metastasis** would be palliated with radiation therapy. (A metastasis is a tumor that results from cancer cells that dislodged from the original or **primary tumor** and spread or **metastasized** to other parts of the body.)

Arturo, an 83-year-old retired architect, was experiencing excruciating pain in his right buttock and thigh. A tumor that metastasized to his lower spine from his lung cancer was encroaching upon nerves, and his pain was not relieved by potent medication. Two weeks after he completed five **radiation treatments**, Arturo noticed a marked improvement. He had less discomfort and his pain was no longer intolerable. He was able to discontinue pain medication after ten days.

Local control, the control of cancer at a particular body site, might be necessary even if the disease cannot be cured. Gladys, a 73-year-old home-maker, has for many years had multiple bone metastases from breast cancer. Several years ago, she had a chest wall recurrence from her breast cancer. Although her metastatic disease was stable, she was felt to be at substantial risk for developing another chest wall recurrence during her lifetime. Such a local recurrence not only would be psychologically devastating for Gladys, but also might cause pain and/or bleeding. Therefore, although her breast cancer could not be cured, Gladys benefited from radiation therapy to the chest wall, which enhanced local control.

Radiation therapy in conjunction with the two main types of **systemic therapy** (chemotherapy and hormonal therapy) often work **synergistically**. This means that the effectiveness of the combination is greater than the sum of the response from radiation therapy and chemotherapy or hormonal therapy when each is given as a sole modality. Many chemotherapy agents are **radiosensitizers**, meaning that they enhance the response of malignant tumors to radiation therapy. Diane (introduced earlier in this chapter) will see optimal tumor shrinkage by the addition of chemotherapy to her radiation therapy.

Radiation therapy can be delivered at the same time as chemotherapy, before chemotherapy has begun, or after chemotherapy has been completed. Despite common misconceptions, radiation treatment is generally kinder and gentler than chemotherapy.

WHY DO YOU NEED RADIATION THERAPY?

Leslie, a lovely 43-year-old puppeteer, underwent a left mastectomy for breast cancer. Leslie feared that she would experience the same unpleasant side effects from radiation therapy that she incurred during chemotherapy. She was amazed at how uneventful radiation therapy to her chest wall actually was.

Systemic therapy is distributed throughout the entire body via the bloodstream, unlike radiation therapy, which is a **local treatment** — meaning it's effective only within the body area where delivered. (Surgery is also a local treatment.) Radiation treatment with chemotherapy and/or hormonal therapy act together upon the primary tumor, whereas the systemic therapy attacks any cancer cells that might have metastasized.

Frank, a 69-year-old plumber with high-risk prostate cancer (cancer that has a high likelihood of extending beyond the prostate gland and/or spreading to lymph nodes and/or bones) is currently receiving hormonal injections and pills that counter the effects of testosterone on his prostate gland. This systemic therapy is intended not only to reduce the volume of his prostate gland and to decrease the number of cancer cells within his prostate, but also to help to **ablate** (eliminate) cancer cells that might have metastasized to his lymph nodes and bones.

Can Frank be cured if his prostate cancer has given rise to microscopic metastases? The possibility that hormonal treatment can eliminate prostate cancer cells that have metastasized and therefore will not be encompassed by the local radiation therapy **portals** (the body area that is treated with radiation) is called **spatial cooperation**.

Radiation therapy is used less frequently to treat benign diseases. Among the non-cancerous entities that are treated with radiation therapy are benign brain tumors, arteriovenous malformations of the brain, pituitary tumors, thyroid-related eye disease (Graves' ophthalmopathy), macular degeneration, keloids, plantar warts, prevention of heterotopic bone formation associated with joint disease, desmoid tumors, and prevention of recurrent blockage of the coronary arteries following angioplasty.

Sean, a 52-year-old disc jockey, underwent radiation therapy to his orbits, the bony sockets where the eyes are located, because of severe thyroid eye disease that did not respond to medication. That was two years ago. Over the weeks and months since radiation therapy, his vision gradually and substantially improved, and the bulging, inflamed appearance of his eyes, which is a common occurrence of the thyroid disorder, resolved.

"When one door of happiness closes, another opens;
but often we look so long at the closed door that
we do not see the one which has opened for us."
– Helen Keller

CHAPTER 2:

WHAT IS RADIATION THERAPY?

DEFINITION OF RADIATION THERAPY

Radiation therapy, also known as radiation treatment, irradiation, and **radiotherapy**, is the use of penetrating beams of high-energy waves or streams of particles to treat disease. Among the sources of these beams are **x-rays, electron** beams, **gamma rays, neutron** beams, and **proton** beams.

HOW RADIATION THERAPY WORKS

Radiation therapy works by ultimately attacking the DNA in the nucleus (center) of a cell. (DNA is the genetic material of cells.) High-energy radiation deposits energy in living tissues through a process called **ionization**, which creates positively and negatively charged particles. The ions cause a chain of chemical reactions within cells. Next, the process of **oxidation** forms highly reactive **free radicals**. These free radicals diffuse (spread) to the nucleus of the cell and cause DNA damage. As the cells die, the clinical effect of radiation is evidenced by the eventual shrinkage of tumors.

Both normal cells and cancer cells are affected by radiation. However, the more slowly dividing normal cells can repair themselves much more efficiently than the rapidly dividing cancer cells. Because the normal cells recover, a therapeutic (or differential) effect is created. Cancer cells generally do not recover, and are therefore eradicated by radiation therapy.

5

What Is Radiation Therapy?

External beam radiation therapy takes place in a treatment room. It is most commonly delivered via a machine called a **linear accelerator**, which delivers penetrating beams of high-energy x-rays or particles called electrons. Cobalt machines deliver another similar form of radiation therapy.

Many facilities have **dual energy linear accelerators**. This means that the linear accelerator has two different high-energy x-ray energies: the first energy is at the lower end of the spectrum of high-energy x-rays and the second energy is at the higher end of the spectrum. (Figure 2-1 shows a photograph of a linear accelerator.)

More superficial tumors, such as head and neck cancers, are best treated with lower energy x-rays and electrons. Unlike x-rays, which penetrate through the body, electrons penetrate to a limited depth. Deep tumors of the chest, abdomen, and pelvis are better treated with higher energy x-rays.

Simulation is the mapping-out session that predates the actual treatment. It takes place in a room that is separate from the treatment room. The machine used in a simulation is called a **simulator**. (See Figures 2-2 and 2-3.)

Often, **CAT scans** are obtained during simulation. A CAT scan is a computerized x-ray that obtains detailed images of the internal structures of a body site. (CAT scans and simulation are discussed in greater detail in Chapter 5.)

For simulation and treatment, you lie on a firm, metal table also referred to as a **couch**. The hardness of the couch prevents you from sagging. This enables your treatment position to be reproduced when you receive your daily treatments.

To ensure that the radiation is delivered most precisely to the site of the cancer, the couch can be slid backward or forward, rotated in a horizontal plane, and raised or lowered. Linear accelerators and simulators have components that can rotate around the patient.

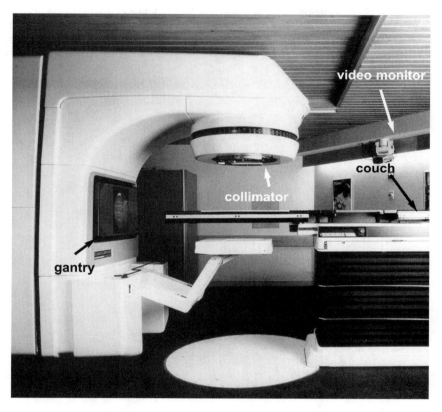

Fig. 2-1. A linear accelerator. It is used for external beam radiation therapy. (Photo © 2001 by Varian Medical Systems. All rights reserved. Used with permission.)

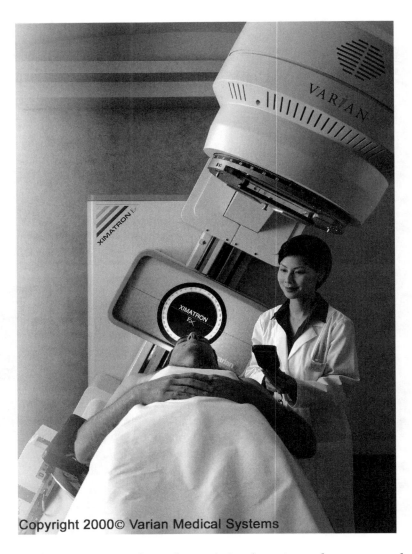

Fig. 2-2. A conventional simulator. A simulator is used to map out the specific body site that will be treated. (Ximatron™ Simulator, Varian Medical Systems. Photo © 2000 by Varian Medical Systems, Inc. All rights reserved. Used with permission.)

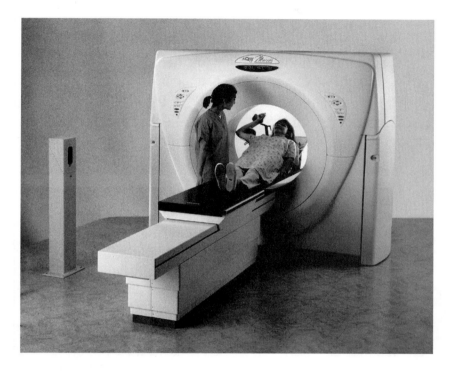

Fig. 2-3. The technologist is positioning a model for a CAT scan simulation of the right breast. (AcQSim™, Philips Medical Systems. Photo © 2001 by Philips Medical Systems. All rights reserved. Used with permission.)

TELETHERAPY

External beam radiation therapy is generated by x-rays, electron beams, gamma rays, neutron beams, and proton beams. External beam radiation therapy is also called **teletherapy**, from the Greek, meaning "therapy from a far distance." This name has been given to external beam radiation therapy because the patient is lying on a treatment table and the source of penetrating beams is relatively far from the patient.

BRACHYTHERAPY

External beam radiation therapy is different from another form of radiation therapy called **brachytherapy**, which, translated from the Greek, means "short distance therapy." Common brachytherapy sources are cesium, iridium, iodine, and palladium. In short, brachytherapy consists of radiation therapy applied directly to the body surface or body cavity, or internally in the form of an **implant** or **seeds**. (Brachytherapy is discussed in Chapter 8.)

X-RAY BEAMS

· X-rays are radiation beams and are defined as low-energy and high-energy.
· Low-energy x-rays are used for diagnostic tests like chest x-rays, mammograms, and CAT scans.
· Low-energy x-rays are also used for **fluoroscopy** (observing the internal body structures by means of x-rays).
· High-energy x-rays are used to treat diseases.

THE RADIATION TREATMENT TEAM

The radiation therapy team consists of a radiation oncologist, the **radiation physicist**, and the radiation therapy **technologists (radiation therapists** or **therapists)**.

The radiation physicist ensures that the radiation treatment machine delivers the correct amount of radiation to the treatment site. Some radiation therapy departments employ a **dosimetrist**, who assists the physicist in developing a radiation treatment plan customized for each patient.

Daily **fractions**, or treatments, of radiation therapy are delivered by the therapists. One of their roles is to position patients on the treatment couch for their daily treatments. They also run the machinery that delivers the radiation.

Some radiation facilities employ a **radiation nurse**, who helps manage a patient's side effects and helps coordinate a patient's care with the other physicians and health care providers who are involved as a team with that patient.

THE RADIATION TREATMENT PLAN

The treatment plan indicates the sizes of the **fields** or areas to be treated, the angles of the radiation fields, and the treatment devices necessary to help deliver the safest and most effective treatment. It specifies the amount of radiation to be delivered to both the cancer and the surrounding normal tissues.

Many treatment plans are developed by a three-dimensional treatment planning computer. **3-D conformal radiation therapy** is a state-of-the-art radiation therapy technique; the radiation beams conform to the shape of the tumor (which I outline on a CAT scan) and spare the surrounding, healthy tissue. (See Figure 2-4 and 2-5.)

DETERMINING FACTORS IN PRESCRIBING TREATMENT

Patients can be treated with brachytherapy alone, external beam radiation therapy alone, or a combination of the two. A patient with localized prostate cancer might receive only external beam radiation therapy because its dose can be adjusted to treat low-, intermediate-, and high-risk prostate cancers effectively.

Low-risk prostate cancer is unlikely to penetrate through the prostate gland or spread to lymph nodes or bones. Intermediate-risk prostate cancer is more likely to do so, but not as likely as high-risk prostate cancer.

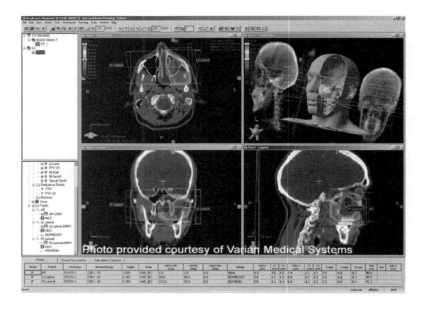

Fig. 2-4. A 3-D treatment plan for cancer of the maxillary sinus. (Photo © 2001 by Varian Medical Systems, Inc. All rights reserved. Used with permission.)

PSA LEVEL
- PSA stands for Prostate Specific Antigen.
- PSA is a chemical that is made by the prostate gland.
- The PSA level is measured from a blood test.
- High PSA levels are found in malignant and benign conditions.

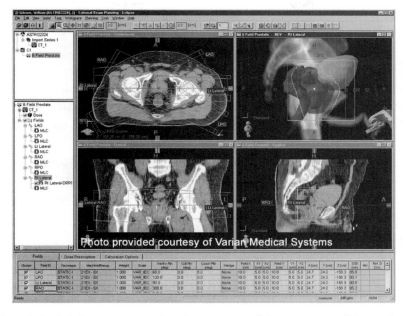

*Fig. 2-5. A 3-D treatment plan for cancer of the prostate. (Photo ©
2001 by Varian Medical Systems, Inc. All rights reserved. Used with
permission.)*

GLEASON GRADE

· This term describes the appearance of thin slices of
prostate cancer when the tissue is observed under
the microscope.

· The ability of cancer to mimic normal prostate
tissue is called **differentiation.**

· Well-differentiated tumors are not aggressive.

· Moderately-differentiated tumors are somewhat
aggressive.

· Poorly-differentiated tumors are very aggressive.

· The lower the Gleason grade, the more well-
differentiated the tumor.

· The higher the Gleason grade, the less well-
differentiated the tumor.

RISK CATEGORIES OF PROSTATE CANCER
· The three categories are low-risk, intermediate-risk, and high-risk.
· Placing a patient into a risk category is based on a combination of the findings on physical examination of the prostate gland, the Gleason grade, and the PSA level.
· A patient is placed in the low-risk category if he has a **nodule** confined to half of one lobe of the prostate, a low Gleason grade, and a PSA level that is less than ten.
· A patient falls into the intermediate-risk category if he has a nodule that involves more than half of one lobe but is confined to the prostate gland, a moderately differentiated tumor, and/or a PSA level between ten and 20.
· A patient falls into the high-risk category if he has any of the following: a nodule that extends outside the prostate gland, a high Gleason grade, or a PSA level greater than 20.

Vincent, a 59-year-old retired military officer, chose to receive the least invasive modality for his intermediate-risk prostate cancer. Thus, he opted for 3-D conformal external beam radiation therapy and declined a brachytherapy prostate seed implant.

Had he chosen to have a prostate seed implant, Vincent still would have required external beam radiation therapy to supplement the dose. A brachytherapy seed implant alone — even though more invasive — would not have been adequate because his cancer was somewhat likely to have extended into the tissues that surround the prostate gland and the radiation dose that the surrounding tissues would receive from an implant would be insufficient.

Although all cancers can spread, some are much less likely to than others. A patient with a substantial risk of the disease's spreading requires a full course of external beam radiation therapy or a shorter course of external beam radiation treatment in addition to a brachytherapy seed implant. Jack, a 63-year-old art dealer with high-risk prostate cancer, decided to have the combination of external beam radiation therapy and a brachytherapy seed implant.

On the other hand, a patient unlike Vincent or Jack, with a low risk of the spread of the disease beyond the prostate gland, can be adequately treated with a brachytherapy seed implant alone. Joe, a 72-year-old semi-retired banker, chose to pursue this option instead of an eight-week course of external beam radiation therapy.

It is not uncommon for systemic therapy, such as hormonal therapy, to precede or accompany prostate seed implants and external beam radiation therapy. Jack and Vincent both began hormonal therapy three months before they embarked on radiation therapy.

Another example of using primary brachytherapy is when a patient is receiving definitive radiation therapy for cervical cancer. Kate, a 75-year-old retired social worker, was well served with a brachytherapy insertion alone, without external beam radiation therapy, because her disease was in a very early stage. Lisa, a 37-year-old school bus driver who had more advanced cervical cancer, required external beam radiation therapy, brachytherapy, and chemotherapy.

EXTERNAL RADIATION THERAPY IS PAINLESS

When I first meet my patients and explain the ABCs of radiation therapy, I emphasize that external beam radiation therapy is a painless, easy procedure, like having a chest x-ray. I assure my patients that during radiation therapy they can breathe normally and will feel no different afterward. The actual treatment takes from one to three minutes, depending on the body site being treated and the complexity of the treatment. Most treatments are delivered daily, Monday through Friday.

External beam radiation therapy is usually delivered in small, daily treatments that build up incrementally over a period that can range from several days to two and a half months, culminating in a grand total dose.

Fractionation (the use of multiple treatments) makes use of the differential effect that radiation has on normal cells, which repair themselves, and cancer cells, which die. Usually one fraction is administered per day, although some diseases are best treated with more than one fraction per day.

15

Two or more fractions per day are separated by at least six hours. The latter application is known as **hyperfractionation**.

Sharon, a 63-year-old medical transcriptionist, received two fractions per day for six weeks for an advanced cancer of the throat. By the last week of her treatment, her tumor had regressed completely.

HOW RADIATION TREATMENTS ARE MEASURED
Daily treatments are measured in units called **rads**, **centigrays**, or **grays**. Standard treatment is delivered at 180 to 200 rads or centigrays per fraction, which is equal to 1.8 to 2 grays, respectively.

The total number of fractions I prescribed for individual patients depends upon the type of disease the person has, as well as on his or her general condition.

Typically, patients change into a gown in a dressing room before they enter the treatment room. For patients who think they will not be able to remain still for treatment because of pain or anxiety, medication may be prescribed.

Josephine, a 74-year-old antique dealer with a diagnosis of breast cancer, had such anxiety she was trembling during her first visit. After taking prescribed medication that diminished her anxiety, she tolerated her sessions well — both the simulation and the first few radiation treatments. After one week, she was no longer nervous, and no longer needed the medication. Relaxation music played in both the simulation and treatment rooms soothed Josephine as well.

Because anxiety can be alleviated by knowing what to expect, I make a point of explaining to patients that positioning them on the treatment table will take five to ten minutes. In that way they know to expect to be in the treatment room for nearly 15 minutes, with only one to three minutes of actual treatment. While no one is in the room with a patient during his or her actual treatment, the therapists monitor patients on a TV screen and via an audio system. During treatment, patients will not see, smell, taste, or *feel* anything.

In the simulation and treatment rooms, beams of red light (laser beams) appear on the walls and the ceiling. These are used to align the patient in a straight plane on the simulator and treatment tables. While the therapists position patients for treatment on the linear accelerator couch, they dim the room lights to enhance the visibility of the laser beams; during treatment the lights are turned back on. Clicking noises made by the mechanical parts of the simulator and treatment machine may be heard, but the radiation beam itself generates no sound.

LASER BEAMS

· Laser beams are light beams that are used to **align**, or straighten, patients on the simulator and treatment tables.
· They are mounted from the ceiling and walls of the simulation and treatment rooms.
· They are not radiation beams.

When patients are set up on the couch, their treatment area is exposed. The rest of their body is draped with sheets or towels, as their dignity is important to the radiation oncology team. After the therapists complete the treatment, patients return to the dressing room.

"The ultimate measure of a man is not where he stands in moments of comfort and convenience, but where he stands at times of challenge and controversy."
-- Martin Luther King, Jr.

CHAPTER 3

YOUR FIRST MEETING WITH THE RADIATION ONCOLOGIST

When new patients arrive for their consult appointment, they are escorted to the consultation/examination room, and the nurse or other staff-person asks several questions. Each patient's blood pressure, pulse, respiration rate, and temperature are recorded along with weight and height. Then each patient is given a gown to change into. The physician reviews their records and x-rays before the first face-to-face encounter.

At the first visit, the physician asks about the patient's present problem, past medical history, past surgical history, current medications, allergies, pertinent family history, social history, and various kinds of symptoms. Then, a full physical examination is performed. Even if a patient is being evaluated for a skin cancer at the tip of the nose, it's customary for a radiation oncologist to perform a comprehensive physical examination. The physician knows that a patient is not just a piece of skin, a breast, a lung, or any other body organ. Every patient is a whole person. Thus, a complete exam is appropriate.

After the examination, the radiation oncologist discusses whether or not radiation therapy is necessary and why. Patients often wish to have family members or significant others present during this consultation.

Additionally, the following should be explained:
- · how radiation therapy will be done,
- · what physical position the patient will be asked to assume during a treatment,
- · what kinds of **immobilization devices** may be necessary,
- · how long the course of treatment is expected to take,
- · how often treatments will be scheduled,
- · how long daily treatments will take, and
- · what simulation, or planning, needs to occur prior to initiating treatment.
- · If any additional lab tests are warranted prior to initiating the course of treatment, this should be discussed as well.
- · The benefits, risks, and alternatives to radiation therapy are also explained.

It is very important that the patient, and his or her loved ones, be given the opportunity to ask questions. There is no such thing as a stupid question. Only when he or she has been apprised of the necessary information and feels that his or her questions have been answered, should the consent form be signed. (See Figure 3-1.)

A patient needs to view his or her radiation oncologist as an ally, not as an adversary. After all, a radiation oncology facility is the last place on earth he or she wishes to be. Having confidence in one's caregivers is essential to a patient's journey into radiation therapy and onto the road to recovery.

During the course of treatment, the radiation oncologist typically sees the patient a minimum of once a week. In addition, making a point of communicating with the referring physicians via consult reports, letters, and phone calls is essential.

Oftentimes, patients will express concerns unrelated to radiation oncology. In such cases, the patient is referred to his or her primary physician, but the issue should never be ignored or dismissed. Illness affects all areas of a person's life and compassion and information must be made available. This is my philosophy with patients, and most physicians and health care providers would agree.

IT IS IMPORTANT TO BE CONFIDENT AND COMFORTABLE WITH YOUR RADIATION ONCOLOGIST

1. Don't be too shy to ask your radiation oncologist if he/she is board certified and uses state-of-the-art equipment (such as dual energy linear accelerators, CAT scan simulation, and 3-D conformal radiation therapy computers).

2. Ask whether your radiation oncologist's facility is certified by the American College of Radiation Oncology, and if he or she attends oncology meetings routinely.

3. Do not feel obligated to remain a patient of any doctor with whom you are not comfortable.

4. You should not be discouraged from seeking another opinion. If you are, you should view this suspiciously and request that your referring physician find another radiation oncologist.

5. In addition to competent clinical skills, compassion and ethical conduct are important qualities in a radiation oncologist. If for any reason you feel that your expectations are not being met, voice your concerns to your referring physician.

CONSENT FOR RADIATION THERAPY

I authorize Dr. Kornmehl and such assistants as she may designate to administer radiation therapy to _____ and to continue such treatments from time to time as he/she deems medically necessary.

I understand that to treat my disease with irradiation, nearby normal tissues and organs may also be directly affected. While every effort is made to decrease these effects, some damage (which most likely will be temporary) may be caused. Occasionally, permanent damage can result.

The effect and nature of this treatment, possible alternative methods of treatment, and the risks of injury despite precautions have been explained to me, and I had the opportunity to question the doctor about these matters. I acknowledge that no guarantees or assurances have been made to me as to the results of the radiation therapy.

I further authorize the tattooing of small marks on my skin to aid in localizing the areas to be treated and understand that these marks will be permanent. In addition, I authorize the taking of photographs by a member of the department staff for purposes of treatment and/or identification only.

Signed:_____

Date: _____   Relationship:_____
                                                   (If other than patient)

Witness:_____
        (Signature only)

I have explained the above treatment to this patient.

_____ M.D.

Fig. 3-1. A sample consent form.

THE CONSENT FORM

The consent form is a legal document. It gives permission for the radiation oncology team to perform treatment.

An informed consent can never be all-inclusive. There are obscure side effects of treatment that might occur, although the probabilities are low. It's similar to getting into a motor vehicle and recognizing that you might have a collision, the vehicle might topple over or catch on fire, you might drive into a pothole . . . If at the time of purchase you had to sign a consent form acknowledging all these remote possibilities, you would probably never want to get into a motor vehicle! You accept the calculated risk, however, because you know that the benefits far outweigh the low risk.

The same is true of radiation therapy. Although many undesirable things might happen, they probably won't, and the benefits of radiation therapy far exceed the risks.

"Not everything that is faced can be changed,
but nothing can be changed until it is faced."
– James Baldwin

CHAPTER 4

RADIATION THERAPY AND YOUR LIFE

Any diagnosis of cancer raises a great many issues that patients become
worried about: life and death, quality of life, disease recurrence in
spite of aggressive treatment, sexual impairment, changes in appearance,
feared loss of bodily and cognitive functions, financial strain — even concerns about transportation to and from radiation therapy. Patients are also
affected by family stress related to a cancer diagnosis. Because treatment
involves the entire human being, not solely the disease, let's examine questions and concerns that normally arise in cancer patients.

LIFE AND DEATH ISSUES

The primary fear for almost all radiation oncology patients is their
mortality. Patients need to acknowledge their worst fears and be realistic
about their prognoses. In doing so, a patient might require the expertise of
a social worker or a psychologist.

Patients who have serious prognoses but are otherwise able-bodied
need a great deal of emotional support. Patients might have a serious prognosis because of a high risk of cancer recurrence, because the cancer could
not be removed completely by surgery, because the disease did not respond
to treatment, or because of known metastases. For patients to heal, their

psychological needs must be addressed. Among the resources that can be utilized are pastoral care, family support, complementary therapy, and anti-depressant or anxiety-reducing medication.

A patient with a serious prognosis benefits from attending a support group. Studies have shown that patients who participate in support groups fare better than their counterparts who do not. Because such groups are made up of peers with similar diagnoses, they facilitate a patient's emotional adjustment to the diagnosis. Support groups help their members develop coping skills or improve those they already have. Susan, a 45-year-old realtor, underwent a stem cell transplant following a modified radical mastectomy for locally advanced breast cancer. While receiving a course of radiation treatments, she expressed several times that her support group was her saving grace.

Admittedly, a support group is not for everyone; therefore, patients who will not attend a group, but who need emotional support, should receive it, either through a private counselor or a pastor, family, or friends. (I encourage such patients to form their own support groups from the circle of friends that they made when they began their cancer treatment odyssey.) Nora, a 44-year-old woman who owns her own commercial cleaning service, was not comfortable speaking about her advanced breast cancer in what she felt was a public forum. She vented to her supportive husband and to her clergyman. Nora also benefited from medication that relieved her anxiety.

I believe in emphasizing to patients that they can and should lead productive lives despite having a serious diagnosis. I have seen many patients outdo their statistical expectations and continue living disease-free for many years. Because you never know who will beat the odds, it is reasonable for people with a cancer diagnosis to live their lives with hope and a conviction that they will outdo the statistics. I stress to my patients the fact that statistics are only a tool. Statistics apply to populations of large numbers of people. One never knows how any individual in that population will fare.

Routine follow-up examinations can detect a recurrence and deal with it appropriately. Additionally, reassurance that no evidence of recurrence exists is something many oncology patients need emotionally, even when they have no physical signs or symptoms of disease. Never forget that time is the best healer. Many of my patients have resumed normal lifestyles and begun to feel as though they are back on an even keel.

LIVING WITH CANCER AND BEATING THE ODDS
In my experience, the most striking example of a patient who outdid the odds is Janine, a retired nurse. She was 65 years old when she was diagnosed as having metastatic breast cancer. Janine was very emotional when I first met her, and rightfully so. She knew that statistically, she had two years to live. She decided to travel to Europe during her remaining time. Eight years later, Janine stopped off to visit me. I was delighted to see her looking so happy, healthy, and radiant. Janine is truly living her life to the fullest.

Patients who have good prognoses but who feel traumatized, distressed, and demoralized by a cancer diagnosis certainly need the previously described psychosocial support. Most of my patients who fall into this category also benefit from a support group, but they should attend one made up of people who share similar prognoses, not who have more guarded prognoses.

For instance, Rebecca, a bright, 40-year-old salesperson, was overwhelmed by her diagnosis of early breast cancer. Yet, she felt optimistic for the first time when she joined a support group.

Although it's natural to worry, worrying creates stress and is therefore counterproductive. More importantly, worrying doesn't drive people to do all they can to change a situation. My suggestion to my patients and their family members is that any time they are concerned, they should let me know. There's usually a way I can provide reassurance. I tell my patients to remind themselves that they are *living* with cancer, not dying from cancer. Mindset is very important.

COMPLEMENTARY THERAPY

Patients may also benefit from complementary therapy. Complementary therapy is not an alternative to standard therapy but is an adjunct to the overall emotional and physical well-being of oncology patients.

Complementary therapy includes: music therapy, art therapy, massage, yoga, reiki, facials, manicures, pedicures, Chinese medicine, herbs, vitamins, magnets, aromatherapy, and other nonstandard therapies. Moreover, you may find more than one of these complementary therapies helpful.

An excellent nonmedical tool is visual imagery occurring during a radiation treatment: you picture in your mind that the radiation is destroying the abnormal cells.

Marilyn, a 71-year-old retired teacher with early breast cancer, swore by magnet therapy. It involves wearing any of the following magnetic devices: necklaces, bracelets, innersoles, kneepads, elbow pads, and corsets. Marilyn taped five-inch circular magnets to her lower back and chest. She slept on a magnetic mattress. Many other forms of magnets are commercially available.

Shannon, a 45-year-old party planner with early stage breast cancer, made a point of going to the spa as often as she could, feeling rejuvenated each time.

LIFESTYLE CHANGES

Another positive step radiation therapy patients can take is to make lifestyle changes, such as discontinuing tobacco and minimizing alcohol intake. To go through cancer-curative therapy and continue to use cancer-causing agents is counterproductive.

Some of my patients make additional positive changes by becoming cancer spokespeople or advocates. The American Cancer Society conducts grassroots training programs. I am also aware of several cancer survivors who have developed or joined chat rooms on the Internet, in lieu of, and in some cases in addition to, attending support groups.

A piece of advice that I gave to Scott, a 34-year-old financial planner with testicular cancer, was that writing an account of his odyssey would probably help others as well as himself. Scott found that writing helped him organize his thoughts. To a large degree the process of writing was also a valuable catharsis.

LIFESTYLE CHANGES AFTER A CANCER DIAGNOSIS
· Tobacco cessation.
· Reduce your alcohol intake.
· Join a cancer support group.
· Join an appropriate chat room.
· Become a cancer spokesperson or advocate
   through the American Cancer Society.
· Write about your feelings in a journal or diary.
· Consider a career change.
· Reduce stressful situations and learn how to
   channel stress constructively.
· Assess what is truly important in your life.

RADIATION THERAPY FOR THE TERMINALLY ILL PATIENT

Radiation therapy has a well-defined role in end-of-life care. A brief course of radiation therapy, usually comprising five or fewer treatments, can enhance the quality of remaining life for a patient whose life expectancy is less than six months.

Among the symptoms that are palliated by radiation therapy are cancer-induced pain, bleeding, and shortness of breath. Radiation therapy is even administered to patients who are receiving **hospice** care. Arturo (the 83-year-old retired architect introduced in Chapter 1) was able to remain at home with hospice care. Depending on the emotional needs of a patient, a hospice program can include pastoral care, family support, and prescribed anti-depressant or anxiety-reducing medication. I believe that the emotional needs of dying patients should be addressed aggressively so they might feel at peace. It is important for such patients and their families to realize that even though radiation therapy won't cure their cancer, the treatments will help relieve symptoms. Despite the fact that oncologists don't have the tools to *cure* every patient, we can nevertheless *help* them.

Let's not lose sight of the fact that the loved ones of terminally ill patients are also suffering. Family members should be encouraged to ask health care providers for whatever help they need. Arturo's wife, for instance, was devastated by her husband's illness and suffering. We steered her in the right direction by advising her to convey her needs to the hospice team. The hospice team had experts trained to help her, even after Arturo passed on.

SEXUALITY AFTER A CANCER DIAGNOSIS

A cancer diagnosis can make an impact on the sex lives of both women and men. This applies equally to heterosexual and homosexual relationships. Problems related to sexuality can stem from psychological as well as physical factors. Be assured that unless one's radiation oncologist advises differently, there is no restriction on sexuality for patients receiving external beam radiation therapy.

For those patients who have had prostate seed implants, inflammation from the procedure causes temporary soreness that might make it unpleasant for a man to engage in intercourse. With prostate seed implants and the administration of other **isotopes**, patients need to wait for the radioactivity to decay to a background radiation level before resuming the physical closeness of sexual intimacy.

Similarly, women who have had vaginal brachytherapy need to wait for their vaginal irritation to subside before they can comfortably resume intercourse. However, a temporary cessation of intercourse is no reason to abandon all forms of intimacy. In fact, closeness and affection are especially important to a patient's sense of self-worth.

The stress of a cancer diagnosis can alienate partners. Stress can also cause distraction that interferes with sexual climaxing. Anxiety about a cancer diagnosis can cause a patient to lose his or her sexual drive. Patients should not be reluctant to discuss these issues with the radiation oncologist, who might be able to offer advice and, if necessary, refer patients to a sex therapist. Olga, a pleasant 49-year-old health insurance administrator, was so preoccupied by her diagnosis of breast cancer that she lost her desire to have sex with her partner. This further exacerbated her anxiety. With the passage of time and with the help of a sex therapist, Olga's sex life returned to normal.

Patients who have had pelvic malignancies, such as rectal cancer, gynecologic cancer, prostate cancer, and bladder cancer, might have physical impairment of sexuality from surgery, chemotherapy, hormonal therapy, and radiation therapy.

Surgery in men as well as women can disrupt the bundle of nerves that enables individuals to achieve orgasm. Again, a sex therapist is able to offer advice on how to compensate for this kind of problem.

Women who have had hysterectomies and/or radiation therapy might feel a narrowing or foreshortening of the vagina. Vaginal dryness and vaginal irritation during intercourse are common occurrences. The use of over-the-counter vaginal lubricants and moisturizers is beneficial. A **vaginal dilator**, a rigid plastic device that resembles a dildo or a large tampon, is very helpful for women who have had radiation therapy to the pelvis. A woman lubricates the vaginal dilator and inserts it into her vagina for several minutes to stretch the tissues and keep them pliable. The dilator is usually used daily or several times per week, as prescribed by the radiation oncologist. Not only does the vaginal dilator help a woman to maintain her sex life, but by keeping the tissues of the vagina from scarring and narrowing, the woman can continue to be examined vaginally.

Changes in position during lovemaking are also helpful.

Women who have had breast surgery and subsequent radiation therapy often experience tenderness in the breast or chest wall. Couples who are passionate and willing to adapt to different positions during intimacy can circumvent this problem. Nancy, a 54-year-old emergency medical technician, found that her irradiated left breast was too tender to let her continue her usual position on the bottom. She switched to the top and was able to enjoy intercourse once again.

Hormonal therapy, especially the kind that is used for prostate cancer, often causes loss of libido, or sex drive. Many men have **erectile dysfunction** that predates their radiation therapy. Ralph, a 73-year-old retired physical education teacher, lost his libido several weeks before his prostate seed implant took place.

While not all sexual problems can be corrected, many can. So be candid with your radiation oncologist, and with your partner, as well.

ECONOMIC ISSUES

A cancer diagnosis can place an economic burden on patients and their families. If the patient cannot work, or can work on a limited basis only, family income inevitably suffers. Additionally, treatment costs, although usually covered by insurance, might not be covered entirely. If the family needs to temporarily relocate while radiation treatments are taking place, additional expenses will be incurred.

Radiation treatments are expensive. If you are uninsured or if you have an exorbitant deductible that is beyond your financial means, a social worker can steer you in the right direction. You might be eligible for Medicaid, or entitled to other benefits that can help defray the costs of radiation treatments. If you are indigent, you might be eligible for charity care. The American Cancer Society is another helpful resource.

As a radiation oncologist, I cannot emphasize strongly enough that I am a physician first and a businessperson second. I have never turned patients away because of financial factors. In most cases, financial arrangements can be made. If your radiation oncologist does not share this philosophy, he or she should not abandon you. Instead, he or she should refer you to another provider who is willing to work with you.

As long as you feel well enough to work while you are receiving radiation therapy, you may do so. In fact, many of my patients continue working while they are receiving radiation therapy and/or chemotherapy. I suggest that patients be candid about their disease and treatment with their employers or supervisors. By communicating their needs, such as time away from work, adjusted hours, or less strenuous assignments, patients are less likely to lose their jobs. I am always writing letters to employers on the behalf of my patients. To the best of my knowledge, not one patient was penalized.

TRANSPORTATION ISSUES

Patients may drive themselves to radiation therapy as long as they feel well enough to do so and do not have a brain **lesion**. If a patient feels so fatigued that he or she might fall asleep behind the wheel, I advise him or her not to drive. The majority of my patients drive for treatments, and many radiation oncology offices have parking spaces designated for their patients.

Still, because radiation therapy usually involves daily treatments Mondays through Fridays for many weeks, some patients find it difficult to commute for their treatments. They might not have friends of family members who can drive them, and they might not be well enough to drive themselves. They might also have pre-existing conditions that render them unable to drive. This was a concern for Arun, an 82-year-old retired engineer with prostate cancer, who had a visual impairment that kept him from driving. Arun was transported to and from his daily treatments via a county bus.

Patients who have brain lesions and who may be at risk for having a seizure while behind the wheel should not drive. This was the case for Eileen, a 49-year-old corrections officer, who had a malignant brain tumor and a history of seizures.

Many counties provide transportation to medical facilities for its citizens. My radiation oncology practice arranges for transportation for those patients who need it because we want our patients to focus on receiving treatment and feeling better, not on how they get back and forth.

Patients should not be reluctant to convey their need for transportation to their practitioners. Patients who need to make their own arrangements might begin by calling the county office on aging. Although illness is not necessarily an aging issue, in many counties, these are the departments that provide transportation.

FAMILY RELATIONS

The dynamics of a family are inevitably affected by a cancer diagnosis. Whether the patient is the parent, grandparent, child, spouse, sibling, aunt, uncle, or cousin, a diagnosis of cancer can affect an entire family. Some families are drawn closer together. Alternatively, a cancer diagnosis can create isolation and a negative change in relationships among family and friends.

Support groups designed for families can benefit family members going through a difficult time. When I find these needs, I direct my patient and his or her family to a social worker, support group, or other means of psychosocial support to help them get back on track.

John, a 58-year-old accountant who underwent surgery for rectal cancer, was torn by the reaction of his wife and daughter to his illness. John was in a high-risk category for cancer recurrence. He required adjuvant radiation therapy and chemotherapy. John and his family were helped greatly by a local social worker. The social worker taught John's wife and daughter relaxation techniques. Thereafter, whenever they began to ruminate about John's disease, John's wife and daughter implemented deep breathing exercises. The family coped well after several weeks.

33

Another family concern is that of hereditary cancers. Patients and their kin are sometimes distressed by the thought that they themselves or others in the family might be carrying cancer-causing genes, or **oncogenes**. To help settle this issue, consider genetic testing. Your radiation oncologist will refer you to a genetic counselor, as needed.

Roberta, a bright, 43-year-old pet shop manager with breast cancer and a strong family history of cancer, was concerned about the future risk of cancer in her three children. She was also worried about her own risk of cancer of her opposite breast and cancer of the ovaries; these cancers are associated with the oncogene for breast cancer. Roberta was referred to a genetic counselor, who helped her make an informed decision about submitting a sample of her blood for genetic testing. Roberta opted to refrain from genetic testing because she was concerned that if she were to test positive for hereditary cancer, she might face discrimination in the future by employers and health insurance companies. Furthermore, Roberta decided that she would not undergo **prophylactic** (preventive) surgery, such as a mastectomy of her opposite breast or removal of her ovaries. She felt that the anxiety a positive test result would generate was something she did not want to bear. Instead, she opted for close follow-up, with physical examinations by her gynecologist and annual mammograms and PAP smears; she will have a colonoscopy, a test to look for tumors of the rectum and large intestine, at age 50.

PHYSICAL AND MENTAL FUNCTIONS

In my experience, a prevailing number of patients worry that after they complete radiation therapy they won't be able to perform the basic bodily functions that all of us take for granted. These functions include moving the limbs such as needed to dress oneself, urinating, defecating (bowel movement), speaking, writing, thinking, eating, drinking, and walking. In many cases there is no need to worry, as these functions are not affected. But be sure to express these concerns to your radiation oncologist, who can address your issues and can refer you to the appropriate specialist, as needed.

Nicholas, a 77-year-old retired bartender with a nonmalignant brain tumor, was worried that his existing difficulties with walking would become more pronounced after he completed radiation therapy. Before he began radiation therapy, Nicholas was referred to a **physical therapist**, who helped him compensate for his leg and arm weakness.

If you are at risk for losing the range of motion of your neck, arms, and legs, your radiation oncologist will also refer you to a physical therapist. She or he can prescribe exercises to keep these muscles and joints limber.

If you have difficulty with your **fine motor skills** such as the ability to button your shirt, dress yourself, or cook for yourself, your radiation oncologist can refer you to an **occupational therapist**. Occupational therapists can teach patients how to compensate for deficits (weaknesses) of fine motor skills. These deficits usually predate radiation therapy and are rarely a consequence of radiation treatment.

If your radiation oncologist anticipates that treatment might affect your speech because of dry mouth, dental problems, or reduced range of motion of your jaw, she or he will refer you to a **speech pathologist** and a dentist.

If your mental acuity were to be affected by radiation therapy, there are existing strategies that would help you to compensate. For example, if you were to develop a problem with your attention span, concentrating on a single task at a time is preferable to doing many things at once. A quiet environment is desirable when you engage in tasks that require intense concentration.

If your memory were to become impaired, you can rely more on visual cues such as sticky notes, calendars, and day planners. An electronic organizer or a handheld tape recorder can be particularly useful. Making lists to help organize and prioritize information, errands, tasks, and other details can aid your recall. You should check off items as you accomplish them.

You should feel free to request the help of your loved ones. They can remind you about appointments and upcoming events. Exercising your mind by playing cards, engaging in stimulating conversation, and reading can be helpful.

Most medical centers offer rehabilitation, called **cognitive retraining programs**. Speech therapists, occupational therapists, **clinical neuropsychologists**, and other rehabilitation specialists conduct these programs.

COSMETIC APPEARANCE

Radiation treatment can result in loss of hair, loss of beard, tooth loss and dental decay, a bulge under the chin called a dewlap, and discoloration of the skin within the irradiated area. That's in addition to cancer surgery having an impact on a patient's perception of her or his own body image.

Patients who have undergone a single or double mastectomy, removal of a testicle, creation of a colostomy or a urinary stoma, amputation of a limb, or neck surgery need to go through not only physical rehabilitation but rehabilitation of self-image.

Convey your concerns to your radiation oncologist. He or she might direct you to "Look Good, Feel Better" programs sponsored by the American Cancer Society. Some "Look Good, Feel Better" programs provide makeovers for women. A makeover can provide to patients the emotional lift they need. Complementary therapy, which I described earlier in this chapter, is also beneficial.

Kathy, a very bright 56-year-old special education teacher with a diagnosis of breast cancer, was feeling bad about her hair loss and weight gain from chemotherapy. She went on a weekend retreat to a spa for breast cancer survivors. The experience left Kathy feeling as though she had recharged her batteries, and her self-image improved dramatically.

"Thou shall not cross bridges before you come to them,
for no one yet has succeeded in accomplishing this."
– Author Unknown

CHAPTER 5

SIMULATION: THE FIRST STEP IN YOUR TREATMENT PLAN

S imulation is a mapping-out session that takes place before any radiation therapy occurs. Think of simulation as a "dry run." The process enables the radiation therapy technologist to know where to locate the radiation therapy beams that will be used for each of your daily treatments.

Like many patients, you might receive treatments over a relatively large area initially, which is reduced in size, or **coned down**, on later occasions during the course of radiation therapy. As the field, or size of each new area changes slightly, more than one simulation session is common. (The particulars of simulation according to body site are discussed in Chapter 6.)

The piece of equipment used in a simulation is called a simulator. (See Figures 2-2 and 2-3.) It has a firm, metal table just like the table of the linear accelerator (shown in Figure 2-1).

You are placed on the simulation table on your back, stomach, or side as determined by your radiation oncologist. If your lesion is on your hand, you might be treated standing up, with your arm outstretched. If your foot is being treated, you might sit on the table with your leg outstretched. If you are positioned on your back, a triangular sponge is placed under your knees or ankles to reduce tension on your lower back and maximize your comfort.

IMMOBILIZATION DEVICES

Many times, the part of your body being treated needs to be immobilized to ensure accuracy. A variety of immobilization devices are available. These devices can keep you from moving during the radiation treatment. and/or reproduce your position for subsequent treatments.

There are several different kinds of immobilization devices. The particular device chosen for you depends upon the body site being treated. If you are being treated for a lesion in the head and neck area, an **aquaplast mask** is commonly used. This mask is made of a perforated plastic material. When the plastic material is heated in a water bath, it becomes flexible and is contoured to your anatomy. It feels like a hot towel on your head and face. As the material cools, it hardens and assumes the shape of your head and facial area. (To see the steps in the construction of an aquaplast mask, please refer to Figures 5-1 through 5-3.)

Chuck is a 51-year-old sanitation worker with a diagnosis of larynx cancer. Throughout his simulation and treatment, an aquaplast mask was used to keep his head and neck in the same position. His head was placed on a special pillow called a **headrest**. (See Figure 5-4.)

Aquaplast strips are prepared in a fashion similar to that of an aquaplast mask. Aquaplast strips are molded around a patient's abdomen, pelvis, and hips, creating immobilization. (See Figures 5-5 and 5-6.)

If your treatments are directed at other parts of your body, you might need an **alphacradle**. It's a support constructed by pouring a liquid chemical mixture into a plastic bag that resembles a garbage bag. (The process is shown in Figures 5-7 through 5-9.) The chemical reaction taking place inside the plastic bag as you lie on it makes you feel its warmth, as if from a heating pad. When you lie on the bag, your body displaces the liquid chemical solution, and the chemical mixture hardens around the periphery of your body into a Styrofoam residue. This forms an impression of your body that fits you perfectly. Dennis, a 49-year-old flight attendant with a diagnosis of pancreatic cancer, lies on his back in an alphacradle for his daily treatments.

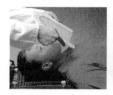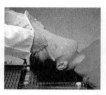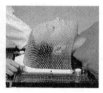

Above, left to right: Figs. 5-1, 5-2, 5-3. Construction of an aquaplast mask to immobilize a patient's head. (Standard disposable Uni-Frame® Masks, MED-TEC, Inc.Photos © 2001 by MED-TEC, Inc. All rights reserved. Used with permission.)

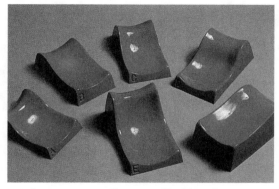

Fig. 5-4. Special treatment pillows, called headrests, are used when the head and neck area is irradiated. (Timo Supports, MED-TEC, Inc.Photos © 2001 by MED-TEC, Inc. All rights reserved. Used with permission.)

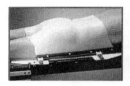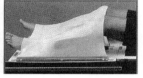

Above: left to right: Fig. 5-5, 5-6. Aquaplast strips to immobilize the patient's abdomen, pelvis, and hips. Hip-Fix is on the left and Pelv-X is on the right. (Hip-Fix® and Pelv-X®,MED-TEC, Inc.Photos © 2001 by MED-TEC, Inc. All rights reserved. Used with permission.)

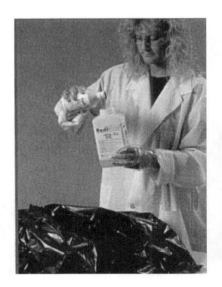

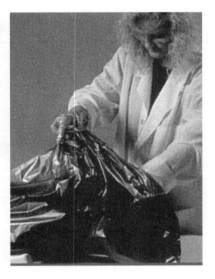

Clockwise from above left:
Figs. 5-7, 5-8, 5-9.
The steps in constructing an
alphacradle (RediFoam™, MED-
TEC, Inc.) are shown in order.
The alphacradle is useful for the
immobilization of many different
body sites. (Photos © 2001 by
MED-TEC, Inc. All rights
reserved. Used with permission.)

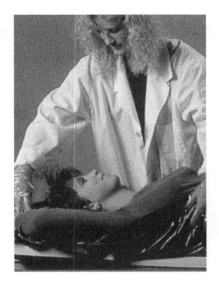

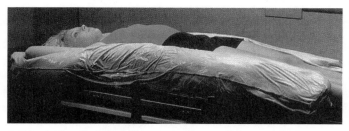

Fig. 5-10. A Vac-Lok Bag™ serves as a mold to reproduce a patient's daily treatment position.(Vac-Lok, MED-TEC, Inc. Photo © 2001 by MED-TEC, Inc. All rights reserved. Used with permission.)

A **Vac-Lok Bag** works on the same principles as an alphacradle, but instead of requiring a chemical reaction, it uses vacuum suction. When you lie on the bag, air is evacuated and Styrofoam pellets within the bag fill in the spaces that surround your body. (See Figure 5-10 for a photo of a Vac-Lok Bag.)

A **breast board** is a rigid, slanted device meant for lying on from the waist up. It has an armrest to support the arm that is kept up and over the head during breast and chest wall radiation therapy. A breast board enabled Elaine, a 71-year-old retired social worker with breast cancer, to lie comfortably for treatments. (Please see Figures 5-11 and 5-12. Figure 5-11 shows how the model in the photo is positioned for radiation treatment.)

Another type of immobilization device is a **lung board.** It has handles, almost like bicycle handles, that you can grasp so that your arms are extended over your head during treatments. (See Figures 5-13 and 5-14.) Daniel, a 79-year-old retired photographer with lung cancer, felt that the handles gave stability to his otherwise shaky arms.

A **belly board** is a rectangular-shaped board made of plastic-like material. A rectangular hole occupies the middle of the board. (See Figure 5-15.) If this is a device your radiation oncologist needs to use for the treatment of your pelvic cancer, you lie on your abdomen on top of this device so that your belly falls into the rectangular hole. This displaces loops of intestine forward, enabling you to receive your treatments in a position easily reproduced each time. Moreover, the likelihood of your developing diarrhea is greatly diminished in this position, which displaces loops of small intestine out of the field.

41

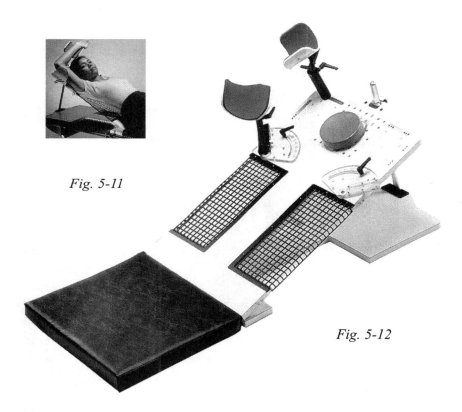

Fig. 5-11

Fig. 5-12

Fig. 5-11 and 5-12. The breast board comfortably immobilizes the patient for radiation therapy to the breast. (MT-250 Composite Breastboard, MED-TEC, Inc. Photos © 2001 by MED-TEC, Inc. All rights reserved. Used with permission.)

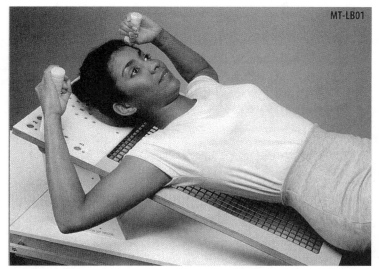

Fig. 5-13

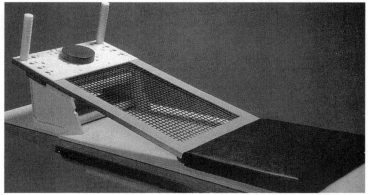

Fig. 5-14

Figs. 5-13, 5-14. The lung board enables the chest treatment position to be reproduced daily. (Lung Board, MED-TEC, Inc.Photo © 2001, MED-TEC, Inc. All rights reserved. Used with permission.)

When abdominal and pelvic fields are treated, the belly board is often used in conjunction with an aquaplast strip, similar to the material used for an aquaplast mask. The strip enhances your immobilization. (See Figure 5-5.)

The belly board and aquaplast strip were useful in Marge's pelvic radiation therapy. A 75-year-old retired nurse's aide, she had been successfully irradiated for breast cancer but received a new diagnosis of cancer of the cervix, unrelated to her breast cancer.

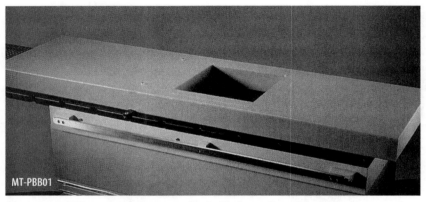

Fig. 5-15. The patient lies on the belly board on his or her stomach. The abdomen is positioned on top of the rectangular hole. This enables the small intestine to fall forward and out of the path of some or all of the radiation beams. (Belly Board™, MED-TEC, Inc. Photo © 2001 by MED-TEC, Inc. All rights reserved. Used with permission.)

Opposite page: Fig. 5-16. Beams from lasers are mounted on the walls and ceiling of the simulation room. These aid the therapist to align the patient on the simulator. Lasers are used in the treatment room for the same purpose. (Stratus™ High-Precision Laser, MED-TEC, Inc. Photo © 2001 by MED-TEC, Inc. All rights reserved. Used with permission.)

ALIGNMENT

After the therapist positions you in your treatment device, he or she straightens or aligns you, using the guidance of the laser beams that are mounted separately from the simulator on the walls and ceiling of the simulation room, together with the aid of an x-ray apparatus that is built into the simulator, called a **fluoroscope**. (See Figure 5-16 for a photo of the laser beams.)

The therapist and radiation oncologist stand behind a booth that protects them from stray radiation. You do not require shielding with a lead apron, as the amount of radiation that you receive from **fluoroscopy** is negligible in comparison to the dose of radiation you will receive from a single treatment.

After your alignment has been ascertained, x-rays emanating from the fluoroscope are used to choose borders for your radiation field. Your skin is marked with a blue marker to indicate the corners of rectangular- or square-shaped fields. X-rays are then taken on the simulation machine. Once your radiation oncologist has approved the films, the field borders are **tattooed.**

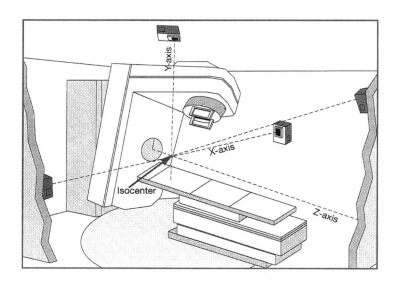

TATTOOS

These are completely different from what people get at a tattoo parlor. Tattoos made for radiation therapy look like dots made with a black ballpoint pen, but are permanent marks made with black India ink. Tattoos never wash away or fade over time. (For a photograph of tattoos, see Figure 5-17.) The benefit of being marked with tattoos is that you don't have to avoid washing away the temporary blue marker dots from one treatment to the next. Tattoos serve as a permanent record of what body area was irradiated should you need a new course of radiation therapy in the future.

Eve, a 45-year-old x-ray technician with breast cancer, was reluctant to have permanent tattoos. Ultimately, she acquiesced. Eve didn't realize how inconspicuous the tattoos would be. She never regretted her decision.

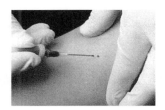

Fig. 5-17. The area of the skin that needs to be tattooed is sterilized with alcohol. The skin is stretched between the technologist's fingers. The technologist gently inserts the needle just under the skin and the India ink tattoos the tiny area. The needle is then discarded. (Steri-Tatt®, MED-TEC, Inc. Photo © 2001by MED-TEC, Inc. All rights reserved. Used with permission.)

OTHER MATERIALS USED FOR SIMULATION

Depending on the area of your body being treated, metal wire might be taped to your skin around tumor masses or scars, so that when I look at the x-rays that we take on the simulator, my attention is directed to the lesion.

Barium might also be gently introduced into your rectum via a plastic tube if I need to identify it on the x-ray films.

You might be given a cupful of barium oral contrast material to drink to fill your small intestines for the x-ray. Barium is a chalky-tasting white or pink liquid.

RADIATION TREATMENT PLANNING CAT SCANS

Many simulations incorporate the use of a CAT scan through the treatment fields. In my office, patients are escorted from the simulation room to the CAT scanner after the fields have been marked on their skin. In some facilities, a CAT scanner is built into the simulator. Either method constitutes state-of-the-art treatment planning.

If your radiation oncologist wants you to have a CAT scan, it takes approximately five minutes to complete. Information from your CAT scan is used by the radiation oncologist, radiation physicist, and dosimetrist to prepare a treatment plan based on your individual anatomy.

*"A healthy attitude is contagious
but don't wait to catch it from others. Be a carrier."*
– Author Unknown

CHAPTER 6

SIMULATION ACCORDING TO BODY SITE

In this chapter, you will take a virtual tour of what radiation therapy simulation entails — according to the body site that is being treated. Bear in mind that every radiation oncologist has his or her unique style of treating patients. The following examples are from my patient files. Medicine is both an art and a science. However, competent practitioners design the treatment fields appropriately. You should skip ahead to the discussion that applies to your own situation.

For those of my patients who anticipate being in pain or feeling anxious during simulation, I prescribe medication(s) to be used half an hour prior to simulation. The same is true for daily treatments. In my practice, relaxation music is played in the simulator and treatment rooms. Music does wonders to reduce the stress from anxiety and pain.

As described in Chapter 5, laser beams mounted from the walls and ceiling are used to properly position each patient on the simulation and treatment tables. The therapist moves the patient to adjust the body to the proper position. Marks are made on each patient's skin with a blue marker or a set of tattoos so the same position can be reproduced each day that radiation therapy occurs.

After your simulation is completed, the therapist takes photographs of your treatment fields. These photos are placed on your chart so the therapists can further identify the field to be treated. For additional identification and to avoid any possibility of treating the wrong patient, a photo of your face is also placed on your chart.

SIMULATION OF THE HEAD

Garrett, a 48-year-old clothing retailer, was diagnosed with a malignant left-sided brain tumor. His simulation entailed the construction of an aquaplast mask, both to immobilize his head during treatment and to enable the outline of the treatment fields to be drawn on the mask, rather than on his scalp. (An aquaplast mask is described in Chapter 5 and shown in Figures 5-1, 5-2, and 5-3.)

Several types of special headrests or pillows are available for use with radiation therapy. (For a picture of these devices, please see Figure 5-4.) Garrett was positioned on his back on the simulation couch, and the appropriate device was chosen according to the position in which his head needed to remain during radiation therapy. In Garrett's case, treatments were done with his head in its normal or **neutral position**. Some patients require that their neck be **hyperextended** or tilted all the way back. Other patients require that their chin be tucked to the chest.

It took ten minutes to make Garrett's mask, align him on the simulation table, and place laser reference marks on his mask. A CAT scan through the field was then obtained. Garrett's CAT scan required injecting contrast material into his veins. The CAT scan took another five minutes.

On Garrett's CAT scan I outlined the area that needed to be treated. The information gleaned from his CAT scan was used by our physicist, who prepared a treatment plan based on Garrett's anatomy. The treatment plan indicated to the technologists what field sizes, what field angles, and what special radiation beam devices we would need to use to give Garrett an effective treatment.

A second simulation took place and simulation x-ray films were taken, following the guidelines of the treatment plan, to verify that what worked on paper would be correct during Garrett's actual treatment. The second simulation took approximately 20 minutes.

The therapists took **beam films** on the linear accelerator after special blocks were prepared to minimize the amount of normal tissue in Garrett's treatment field. (The preparation of blocks is discussed later in this chapter. See Figures 6-7 and 6-8.) Once I approved the beam films, which verified that the radiation beams would be hitting the correct target, Garrett began his radiation therapy.

BEAM FILMS
During the course of the radiation treatments, weekly beam films (also known as **port films**) are taken on the linear accelerator to verify ongoing quality assurance:
· These are compared to the x-rays obtained at the time of your simulation.
· From the beam films, the radiation oncologist can determine if the blocking is correct and if the radiation beam is treating the intended area of your body.

DEVICES THAT DETERMINE THE SHAPE OF THE RADIATION BEAM
Blocking is devised by your radiation oncologist to give a margin of normal tissue around your tumor and/or its draining lymph nodes. The block is shaped to the tumor to exclude as much normal tissue as possible from the treatment beam, although your tattooed field might be shaped like a square or a rectangle. This measure helps to limit side effects.

Customized lead alloy blocks are mounted on an acrylic tray. The tray is slid into the **collimator** (a component of the treatment machine that narrows the radiation beam by shaping it into a rectangle or a square) of the linear accelerator or cobalt machine. (See how blocks are inserted into the collimator in Figure 6-8.) Some linear accelerators have **multileaf collimators**. These are computer-driven blocking devices that work on the same principle as customized blocks.

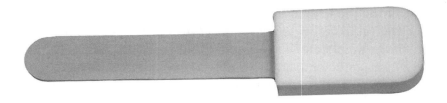

Fig. 6-1. Bite block. The spongy end is inserted into the patient's mouth. It separates the upper and lower jaws. Therefore, normal tissue is moved out of the radiation field. (Bite®, Sage Products, Inc. Photo © 2002 by Sage Products, Inc. All rights reserved. Used with permission.)

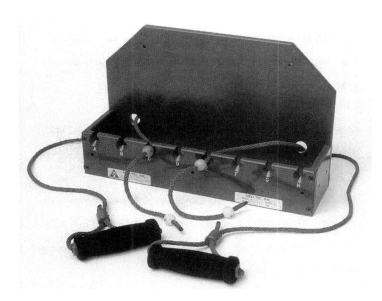

Fig. 6-2. Jump rope to retract the patient's shoulders. The base plate is positioned against the patient's heels, and the patient pulls on the jump rope handles. (Shoulder Retractors, MED-TEC, Inc. Photo © 2001 by MED-TEC, Inc. All rights reserved. Used with permission.)

HEAD AND NECK SIMULATION

Most of the same principles that are described in the section on simulation of the head apply to simulation of the head and neck. Bill, a 73-year-old retired tool and die machinist with a diagnosis of cancer of the right salivary (parotid) gland, underwent surgery to remove the tumor. He was at high risk for having cancer grow back in the **tumor bed** (the tissue that surrounds the site from which a tumor has been removed) and the lymph nodes of his neck, a risk based on certain features of the tumor that were identified when it was studied under a microscope. Therefore, he required post-operative radiation therapy.

Bill was placed on his back on the simulation couch. If Bill had any lumps or enlarged lymph nodes, which he didn't, I would have delineated these with metal wire so that the area of interest might be identified on x-ray films. Metal wire was taped onto his surgical scar.

Bill's head and neck simulation required the use of a **bite block**, a sponge-like device that is attached to a tongue blade. It kept Bill's mouth open during radiation therapy, thereby keeping his lower jaw and tongue out of the radiation therapy field as much as possible. (Figure 6-1 shows a picture of a bite block.)

To pull Bill's shoulders down and out of the radiation therapy field, he was given a device that looks like a jump rope. He held onto the jump rope with his hands and pulled it against his heels. His back remained in its original position, as only his shoulders shifted. (For a picture of this device, please see Figure 6-2.)

Using the fluoroscope built into the simulator for guidance, I identified a rectangular-shaped field for treatment and outlined the borders of that field on Bill's mask with blue marker.

The field of Bill's lower neck extended lower than the bottom edge of his aquaplast mask. Therefore, he needed tattoos of the lower neck field borders. X-rays of the fields were taken.

Bill next underwent a CAT scan through the head and upper neck fields. The area that needed to be treated was outlined on Bill's CAT scan.

Simulation According to Body Site

Chest Simulation

Livia, a 56-year-old gospel singer with a diagnosis of lung cancer, required radiation therapy to her chest. Due to severe shortness of breath, Livia needed oxygen. She carried a portable tank. Around her head, she wore a thin, clear tube that conducted the oxygen from her tank into her nose.

Because of the location of her tumor, she was positioned on her back. Her arms were extended over her head with a device called a lung board. (To see what a lung board looks like, please refer to Figure 5-14.)

In addition, an alphacradle was constructed to keep Livia's position reproducible every day. (A picture of an alphacradle appears in Figure 5-9.)

Livia had a hacking cough that could have made it difficult for her to remain motionless, so I prescribed a cough suppressant for her. Livia's oxygen tank presented no obstacle to her daily treatments, as it was placed next to her on the treatment table.

Using the guidance of the fluoroscopy component of the simulator, the therapist and I localized a rectangular-shaped field on her chest. Field borders were outlined on her skin with blue marker. These borders and the center of the field were tattooed. Marks to align Livia in a straight plane were also tattooed on her chest. This procedure took approximately 20 minutes.

Livia's chest simulation incorporated the use of a CAT scan, for which she received an injection in her veins of contrast material. The CAT scan took another five minutes. She tolerated the procedure very well.

Inga, a 64-year-old optician, needed radiation therapy for a tumor of the esophagus. She was positioned in the same way as Livia and, similarly, needed a CAT scan for treatment planning purposes. She was given a thick, chalky barium paste to swallow during her simulation. This material helped us to visualize Inga's esophagus and to identify where in her esophagus the obstructing tumor was located.

After Livia's and Inga's simulations, I outlined on each of their CAT scans the area that needed treatment.

Livia and Inga also had a second simulation to verify that what worked on paper would be correct during an actual treatment. X-ray films were taken. The second simulation took 15 minutes.

ABDOMINAL SIMULATION

Richard, a 53-year-old carpenter who underwent partial removal of his stomach for cancer of the stomach, required post-operative radiation therapy to his upper abdomen. Part of his stomach and its draining lymph nodes were encompassed in the area to be treated.

Because he'd already had a surgical procedure and was undergoing post-operative radiation therapy, the first step of his simulation was to obtain a **scout film** on the simulator, to identify the **surgical clips** that Richard's surgeon had placed in the area where the tumor was situated.

Surgical clips resemble tiny metal pellets or staples. Surgeons often place clips around tumors that cannot be removed, as well as around the tumor bed. The clips are visible on x-rays and they help the radiation oncologist design a custom shaped treatment field.

The scout film enabled us to clearly visualize this area, because the clips would be obscured by the barium that Richard would be drinking to provide the contrast for the simulation x-rays. Approximately 30 minutes after drinking a cupful of barium, Richard was once again placed on the simulation table on his back.

Because barium tends to cause constipation, Richard was advised to take two tablespoons of Milk of Magnesia and drink copious fluids during the rest of the day following his simulation.

An alphacradle was constructed to ensure that Richard's position on the treatment table would be reproduced each day. (See Figure 5-9 for a photo of an alphacradle.) Additionally, his arms were extended over his head with the use of a lung board. This measure moved his arms out of the path of the radiation beams. (See Figure 5-14.) After x-ray films were taken and approved, the rectangular-shaped field was marked and tattooed on Richard's abdomen. Then he underwent a CAT scan. The entire simulation took 45 minutes.

Christina, a 74-year-old church secretary, underwent surgery to remove a malignant tumor from the left side of her colon. Because the tumor penetrated through the wall of her bowel, she required post-operative radiation after her surgical wound healed. Christina's simulation took 45 minutes.

She went through the same procedures that Richard did, except that she was positioned on her right side so that the left side of her body was elevated. To reproduce Christina's daily position on the treatment table, we fashioned an aquaplast strip. (See Figure 5-5.)

Under fluoroscopic guidance, Christina's alignment was ascertained and marked on the aquaplast strip. Several alignment tattoos were made on her skin. Field borders were chosen, also with the guidance of the fluoroscope. The radiation therapy field center and borders were marked on the aquaplast strip. A CAT scan was then obtained, taking an additional five minutes.

On Richard's and Christina's CAT scans, I outlined the area that each needed to have treated.

PELVIC SIMULATION

Marianne, a 79-year-old retired dental office manager with a diagnosis of bladder cancer, required radiation therapy to her pelvis. She was given a cupful of barium contrast to drink so that I would be able to identify her small intestines on x-ray films. Approximately 30 minutes later, simulation began.

I instilled contrast material into her bladder via a pediatric-sized **catheter** (a flexible, hollow tube), under sterile conditions. This measure enabled us to visualize Marianne's bladder on simulation x-ray films.

Doris required radiation therapy for rectal cancer. A 52-year-old school psychologist, Doris had a surgical procedure and needed post-operative radiation therapy to eradicate any cells that might not have been removed at the time of her operation. A scout film was obtained to identify surgical clips that Doris's surgeon placed where the tumor was situated. The scout film enabled us to clearly visualize this area, because once Doris drank barium, the clips were obscured.

It is standard practice to treat the scar between the buttocks where Doris's rectum used to be. At the time of her operation, the tissues that surrounded her rectum were stitched together, and a colostomy was constructed. During her simulation, I taped a metallic marker on the scar so it would be identified on simulation x-rays.

Dominic, a 70-year-old retired fire fighter, required radiation therapy for cancer of the anus. Dominic's tumor protruded from his rectum, so metallic wire was placed around the tumor and taped into place, enabling me to visualize the location of the tumor on a simulation x-ray.

For women patients, I introduce a smooth, tampon-shaped, plastic device called a **vaginal marker** into the vagina so the vagina might be identified on the x-ray. In male and female patients who have not undergone surgical removal of the rectum, I instill barium into the rectum via a soft, rubber catheter, so that it might be identified on the x-rays that we obtain on the simulator.

The simulations of Marianne, Doris, and Dominic were performed by having each lie face down, utilizing a belly board. The therapist constructed a customized aquaplast strip for immobilization. (Please see Figures 5-5 and 5-15 for a picture of these devices.)

To be sure that each patient was lying straight, we used the laser beams, as well as the fluoroscopic guidance of the simulator to ascertain alignment. The therapist tattooed the alignment marks. I chose square- or rectangular-shaped field borders under fluoroscopy for each individual, and blue marker was used on both the buttocks and on the sides of both hips to outline the fields. Tattoos then marked these borders, each patient's alignment, and the center of each field. A CAT scan was performed through the treatment field on the buttocks, which took approximately five minutes for each patient. After their simulations were completed, Marianne, Doris, and Dominic were advised to take two tablespoons of Milk of Magnesia and drink copious fluids for the day to avoid constipation from the barium drink.

Vincent, the 59-year-old former military officer discussed in Chapter 2, underwent 3-D conformal radiation therapy for prostate cancer. For his simulation, Vincent was placed on his back and his stockinged feet were taped together to help limit his movement during the simulation and treatment. An alphacradle was constructed to reproduce his position for daily treatments. Vincent's alignment was checked under fluoroscopy to make sure that he was lying in a straight plane. His alignment was then tattooed.

Under fluoroscopic guidance, a point was chosen near the pubic bone, which is the bone that lies in front of the pelvis. This point was tattooed on Vincent's skin as a reference point.

Before the CAT scan and before each daily treatment, Vincent was asked to empty his bladder because the prostate gland changes position with a full bladder. An empty bladder keeps the prostate's position consistent. After x-ray contrast was introduced into his bladder and into his urethra — the organ that connects the bladder to the penis — a CAT scan was obtained through Vincent's prostate gland.

The procedure of instilling contrast into the bladder and urethra is called a **cystourethrogram**, and it takes less than five minutes. During this procedure, the patient's penis is sterilized with iodine. Liquid contrast material is infused into the bladder via a pediatric-sized catheter, which is lubricated and introduced into the patient's penis and positioned in the bladder. The catheter is then withdrawn approximately one inch to situate it in the penis. Additional contrast material is instilled into the catheter until it is seen to be dribbling out of the penis. At that time a cushioned clamp is placed around the penis to keep the contrast material from dribbling out completely. A cystourethrogram is slightly uncomfortable but it is not painful.

Vincent's simulation lasted 20 minutes. The cystourethrogram helped me identify both the top and the bottom of Vincent's prostate gland. (For a picture of an example of a cystourethrogram, please see Figures 6-3 and 6-4.)

On the CAT scan, I outlined the area that needed to be treated. (Figure 2-5 shows an example of a treatment plan.)

A second simulation took place on the simulator to verify that what worked on paper would be correct when Vincent was treated. X-rays (simulation films) were taken. Vincent's second simulation took 20 minutes.

Tom, a 30-year-old computer software developer, required radiation therapy to his abdominal and left pelvic lymph nodes after testicular cancer caused the removal of his left testicle. I anticipated a substantial amount of scattered radiation to Tom's remaining testicle, so a **clamshell shield** was used. (Figure 6-5 shows a picture of this device.) Tom applied the clamshell shield himself to minimize any pinching of the skin of the scrotum.

Pedro, a sweet six-year-old boy with leukemia, needed irradiation of his testicles to eradicate leukemia cells. Therefore, his testicles were not shielded. Pedro's testicles were propped up and away from his pelvis with a square-shaped piece of Styrofoam. Pedro's penis was gently taped up against his upper pelvis and out of the field. I devised an appropriately shaped lead block, called a cutout, to shield the normal, surrounding tissues. The cutout was suspended from the linear accelerator and did not touch Pedro's skin. His simulation took ten minutes.

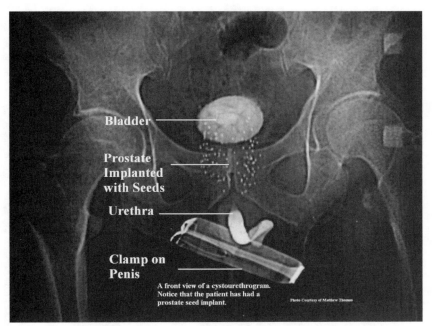

Fig. 6-3. A front view of a cystourethrogram. Notice the contrast in the bladder and urethra, giving them the whitish color. This patient had a prostate seed implant. (Photo © 2002 by Matthew Thomas. All rights reserved. Used with permission.)

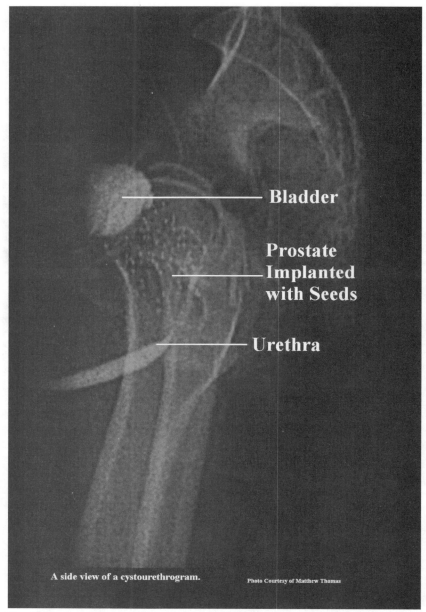

A side view of a cystourethrogram.

Fig. 6-4. A side view of a cystourethrogram. (Photo © 2002 by Matthew Thomas. All rights reserved. Used with permission.)

SKIN LESION SIMULATION

A simulation of the skin depends on the body part that is being treated. For example, Patricia, an 83-year-old nursing home resident, required treatment for a lesion on the left side of her scalp. Patricia was placed on the radiation treatment table with her head turned to the right, a position that best exposed the lesion to the radiation therapy beam.

Felix, an 89-year-old retired sailor, had skin cancer on the back of his scalp. He was placed on his stomach.

Peggy, an 85-year-old retired clerk, had skin cancer on her nose. She was placed on her back and her head was positioned straight.

For Patricia, Felix, and Peggy, an aquaplast mask was used. Such a device is commonly used during radiation therapy for skin lesions of the facial and head area. The areas that needed treatment were delineated with a blue marker. With Peggy's lesion of the nose, marking the area would have been unsightly. Therefore, we marked Peggy's mask based on how the laser beams indicated accurate alignment. These marks were then used to reproduce Peggy's position for daily treatment.

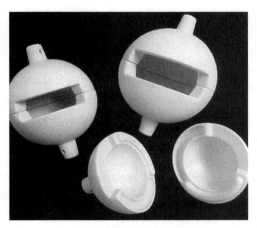

Fig. 6-5. Clamshell shield. The 2 halves are placed by the patient around his testicle. (Testicular Shield, MED-TEC, Inc. Photo © 2001 by MED-TEC, Inc. All rights reserved. Used with permission.)

Wilbur, an 82-year-old former owner of a liquor store, had a basal cell skin cancer on his back. He was placed on his stomach on the table, and an alphacradle (Figs. 5-7, 5-8, 5-9) was constructed to reproduce Wilbur's daily position.

Bertha, a 76-year-old retired seamstress, had a skin cancer on her chest. She was positioned on her back, and an alphacradle was constructed for the purpose of immobilizing her and reproducing her daily position.

Larry, a 68-year-old karate instructor, had skin cancer on the side of his right shoulder. He was placed on his left side, and an alphacradle was constructed to reproduce his position for daily treatments.

Skin cancers of the arms, hands, legs, and feet are treated in whatever position is optimal. For example, Byron, a 64-year-old advertising agent, had a skin cancer on his right shin. Byron was placed on his back, and his right leg was immobilized with an alphacradle. If the lesion had been on the back of his leg, Byron would have been placed on his stomach, and the alphacradle would have been constructed using the same principles as used for the front of his leg.

Albert, an 83-year-old retired railroad worker, had a skin cancer on the back of his right hand. The optimal treatment position was to have him stand with his right arm stretched out on the treatment table. An alphacradle was used to reproduce Albert's daily treatment position.

These skin simulations took no longer than ten minutes each. All of my patients tolerated the procedure well. For their daily treatments, **bolus** material was placed over their treatment areas.

Bolus is a rubbery, smooth, nearly transparent, flexible material. It acts as an artificial skin layer, enabling the radiation beam to build up to its maximum dose just underneath. The immediately underlying skin then receives the full dose of radiation, instead of being spared. (To see what bolus material looks like, refer to Figure 6-6.)

BREAST AND CHEST WALL SIMULATION

Liz, a 39-year-old cashier, underwent a right lumpectomy for early stage breast cancer. She required radiation therapy to the right breast only.

Genevieve, a 51-year-old nanny, underwent a modified radical mastectomy for locally advanced cancer of the left breast. Because four out of six axillary (underarm) lymph nodes tested positive for cancer cells, Genevieve needed chemotherapy first, followed by radiation therapy to her left chest wall, to the lymph nodes in her lower left neck, and to the remaining lymph nodes in her left axilla.

For Genevieve and Liz, their placements were similar. Each lay on her back on a breast board on the firm simulation table. (See Figure 5-12.) The arm on the side that was being treated was placed over her head. The breast board served as an immobilization device that helped to reproduce the position for each woman's daily treatment. After fluoroscopic guidance ascertained that Liz's and Genevieve's alignments were in a straight plane, I defined field borders for the rectangular-shaped fields. Liz's simulation took 15 minutes; Genevieve's, 25 minutes.

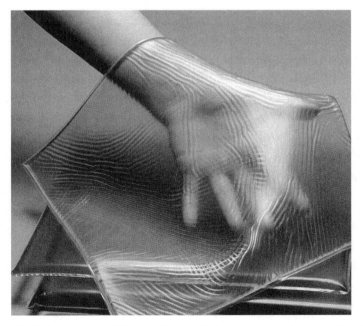

Fig. 6-6. Bolus material is used when it is necessary to give the skin a full dose of radiation therapy. (Bolus, MED-TEC, Inc.Photo © 2001 by MED-TEC, Inc. All rights reserved. Used with permission.)

SIMULATION ACCORDING TO BODY SITE

Because Genevieve's radiation therapy would treat the supraclavicular fossa (lower neck) and extend to the top of her axilla (underarm), these fields were mapped out first. Simulation x-rays were taken, and I drew customized blocks on her films. The blocks were prepared using a special device called a block cutter. (For a picture of such a device, please see Figure 6-7.) The borders and center of the supraclavicular fossa and axillary fields were then tattooed.

After Genevieve's supraclavicular fossa and axillary fields were mapped out, the simulation couch was turned slightly to the left so the top of the chest wall fields would match up with the bottom of her supraclavicular fossa and axillary fields. The amount of lung and heart in the chest wall field was checked under fluoroscopy to make sure that it was not excessive. Once I was satisfied, Genevieve had a CAT scan throughout her chest wall. Our physicist prepared a treatment plan based on Genevieve's anatomy using the information from the CAT scan.

Liz's simulation of the breast entailed the same procedures. However, the fields of the lower neck lymph nodes and the lymph nodes of the underarm were excluded.

Both women underwent a second simulation: for Liz, of her breast, and for Genevieve, of her chest wall. The repetition verified that what worked on paper would be correct when each woman was treated. The second simulation took no longer than 20 minutes. In Liz's case, solder wire was taped around her breast; for Genevieve, her mastectomy scar was delineated with solder tape. When x-rays were taken, I was able to draw blocks on the films to spare as much normal tissue as possible. The borders of Liz's breast field and Genevieve's chest wall field were subsequently tattooed.

Before their treatments began, we obtained beam films on the linear accelerator to verify that the radiation beams would treat the correct body sites.

I generally prescribe an extra radiation dose to the tumor bed, as the area of the breast from which the tumor was removed has a higher risk of harboring cancer cells than other parts of the breast. Similarly, a mastectomy scar is more likely to harbor cancer cells than other parts of the chest wall. The smaller treatment area is called a **boost** or a **cone down**.

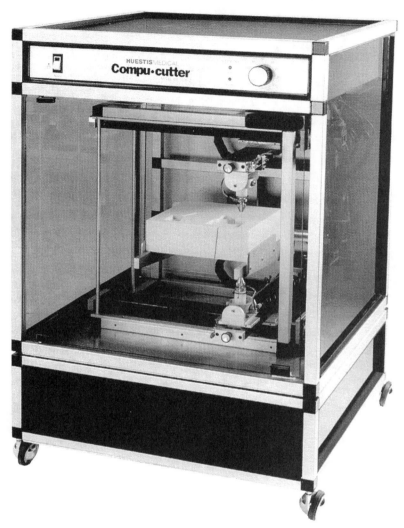

Fig. 6-7. Block cutting machine. A wedge of Styrofoam is cut with a jigsaw, according to the shape of the blocks that the radiation oncologist draws on the simulation x-ray film. The interior of the Styrofoam is pushed away by the therapist. The exterior is then mounted on a perforated acrylic tray. The therapist then pours heated, liquefied lead alloy into the mold formed by the Styrofoam. Once the lead alloy solidifies, the therapist removes the Styrofoam mold.
(Compu•Cutter®, Huestis Medical. Photo © 1996 by Huestis Medical. All rights reserved. Used with permission.)

When Liz was ready to begin her cone down to the tumor bed, and Genevieve was ready to undergo a boost to her mastectomy scar, I defined their cone down areas.

Liz's surgeon had inserted metallic surgical clips into the cavity where her breast tumor was removed. The clips were identified on an x-ray that the therapist took on the simulator, and the cone down treatment area was well defined. In Genevieve's case, I drew the cone down field on her skin with blue marker.

Their respective breast and chest wall boosts were delivered with an electron beam. A customized lead cutout defined the shape of the field. Each field was marked with a purplish-red food-coloring derivative. Tattoos were not used in this situation. Because the food-coloring derivative stains fabric, I told Liz and Genevieve to wear either dark clothing or clothing that had little value during the brief time that they needed to retain the food-coloring derivative marks. Each woman was able to shower but needed to keep her back to the water. The marks were touched up every day by our therapists.

SIMULATION OF THE ARMS AND LEGS (EXTREMITIES)

Mary, a 47-year-old waitress, underwent surgical removal of a soft tissue sarcoma from the muscles of the back of her right forearm. Mary needed post-operative radiation therapy to eradicate any cells that might have been left behind.

An alphacradle was constructed to reproduce Mary's position for daily treatment. She was best served by lying on her stomach on the simulation table, with her right arm stretched in front of her. For her daily treatments she assumed the same position. Mary's simulation took 30 minutes.

After an alphacradle was constructed of Mary's upper body, including her outstretched right arm, I taped metallic wire onto her surgical scar so that it might be visualized when x-rays were taken. Blue marker was used to identify the treatment borders of the rectangular-shaped fields. The field borders and field center were tattooed, and after a contrast dye was injected into Mary's veins, a CAT scan was done throughout the treatment fields.

I then outlined on the CAT scan the area that needed to be treated. Our physicist, who used the information from the CAT scan, prepared a treatment plan based on Mary's anatomy.

Before her treatment began, beam films were obtained on the linear accelerator to verify that the radiation beams were hitting the correct target.

Bolus material was placed over the surgical scar to enhance the radiation so that Mary's skin would receive a full dose of radiation; otherwise, the radiation beam would spare the surface of her skin and the surgical scar would be underdosed.

Clayton, a 69-year-old crossing guard, had pain in his left hip because of a bone metastasis from kidney cancer. He wanted to continue to work, but pain made it difficult to walk and stand. Because pain control was important, he chose to receive radiation therapy to his left hip.

With Clayton lying on his back on the simulator couch, an alphacradle was constructed to keep his position reproducible for daily treatment. Fluoroscopic guidance verified that his alignment was straight. Field borders were chosen under x-ray guidance, and the square-shaped field was outlined on the skin of his left groin area. X-ray films were taken of the field from the front and the back.

After I approved his films, the field borders were tattooed. I devised customized blocks to spare as much healthy tissue as possible. His simulation took 15 minutes. Before Clayton's treatment began, beam films were taken to verify that the radiation beam was hitting the correct target.

BONE SIMULATION

Simulation usually takes 20 minutes when performed on bones, such as the skull, **vertebral bodies** or **vertebrae** (spine bones), ribs, and bones of the arms, legs, shoulders, and hips.

Ben, an 86-year-old retired wine distiller with a diagnosis of metastatic cancer of the prostate, had simulation of the bones of the vertebral bodies of his neck. I prescribed his radiation therapy for pain control. Ben was placed on his back on the simulation couch. An aquaplast mask was constructed, and a headrest was used to support his head and neck. (See Figures 5-1 through 5-4.) Using the laser beams and fluoroscopic guidance, Ben was aligned in a straight plane. Blue marker on Ben's mask outlined the rectangular-shaped fields that I chose under fluoroscopic guidance.

X-ray films were obtained, and I drew customized blocks on the films. Then, beam films were obtained on the linear accelerator before Ben's treatment began.

Dorothy, a 74-year-old homemaker with metastatic lung cancer, required radiation therapy to control pain from a lesion that was eroding several vertebrae in her lower back. Dorothy was placed on her back on the simulator. An alphacradle was constructed by the therapist to reproduce her daily position. (See Figures 5-7 through 5-9.) Under fluoroscopic guidance and using the laser beams, we ascertained Dorothy's alignment so that she would be lying in a straight plane. I chose field borders under fluoroscopic guidance. Blue marker was used to mark the outline of the rectangular-shaped fields. After we obtained x-ray films, I drew customized blocks on the films. The field borders and the field center were subsequently tattooed on her chest and abdomen by the therapist. Beam films were obtained from the front and back on the linear accelerator before Dorothy's daily treatment began, to verify that the proper area would be irradiated.

Dave, a 68-year-old retired printer, had painful right lower back rib lesions secondary to multiple myeloma. Dave was placed on his stomach, the position that best exposed the affected ribs. An alphacradle was constructed to reproduce Dave's daily position. Under fluoroscopic guidance and using the laser beams, his alignment was ascertained so that he would be lying in a straight plane for his treatments. Blue marker was used to mark the outline of the rectangular-shaped field. A simulation film was obtained to record the field borders and field center. These borders and the center were subsequently tattooed on his back. Dave's rib lesions were treated with an electron beam.

SIMULATION OF THE MANTLE FIELD (LYMPH NODES OF THE NECK, UNDERARMS, AND CHEST)

Radiation therapy for Hodgkin's disease is classically delivered through a field called a **mantle** field. The mantle field includes lymph nodes of the neck, axillae (underarms), mediastinum (lymph nodes inside the chest cavity), and hilum (also lymph nodes inside the chest cavity).

Matthew is a 50-year-old graphic designer with early stage Hodgkin's disease. Matthew was placed on his back, and with the support of a headrest, his head was extended as far back as it could go. (For a picture of such a headrest, please see Figure 5-4.) Solder wire was taped around the enlarged lymph nodes of the left side of his neck so I would be able to identify them when an x-ray film was taken.

An aquaplast mask was constructed to keep Matthew's head immobilized and to reproduce his position for his daily treatments. He was asked to place his hands on his hips, assuming what is called the **akimbo position**, and an alphacradle was constructed from his shoulders down to his hips. (See Figures 5-1 through 5-3 and Figures 5-7 through 5-9 to see photos of these devices.)

Under x-ray guidance, Matthew's alignment was ascertained so he would lie in a straight plane. Field borders were chosen. Upper border marks were placed on the mask; lower border marks were made on his skin with blue marker, and the corners and the center of the field were tattooed on his chest. X-ray films were taken of the field from the front and back. His mantle simulation took 20 minutes.

On his x-ray films I drew customized blocks. These were subsequently prepared on the block cutter by the therapist. (See Figure 6-7.) These lead blocks were suspended from the linear accelerator — not placed on Matthew. (Figure 6-8 shows how the therapist places the blocks.) The blocks shaped the field, thereby excluding as much normal tissue as possible.

Matthew was given an injection of contrast before his CAT scan was performed. From the CAT scan data, our physicist obtained information about Matthew's anatomy. Our physicist then determined what doses the various areas of the mantle field would receive, such as the nodes in his upper neck and the lymph nodes in the middle of his neck, lower neck, chest, underarms, and spinal cord. Before beginning radiation therapy to the mantle field, Matthew underwent beam films on the linear accelerator. He began treatment once I approved these films.

SIMULATION OF THE SPLEEN AND ABDOMINAL LYMPH NODES FOR HODGKIN'S DISEASE

Matthew also required a simulation of his spleen and abdominal lymph nodes. The lower border of his mantle field was identified so it could be matched under x-ray guidance with the top border of his spleen and abdominal lymph node field. This way, an overlap of the spinal cord was avoided.

The rest of the field borders were chosen under fluoroscopic guidance. It was ideal to use the same alphacradle already constructed for Matthew's mantle field and to keep him in the same position. Matthew's arms remained in the akimbo position. However, treatment of the spleen and abdominal lymph node fields did not require his neck to be extended backward so we didn't use his aquaplast mask. X-ray films were obtained from the front and back and the field borders and field center were tattooed on his abdomen.

Matthew was subsequently given contrast material in his veins for a CAT scan, which yielded information for our physicist to develop a treatment plan based on Matthew's abdominal anatomy. The simulation took 20 minutes.

I drew customized blocks on Matthew's films. Before radiation treatment to the spleen and abdominal lymph node fields began, beam films were obtained on the linear accelerator. Matthew's treatment commenced once I approved the beam films.

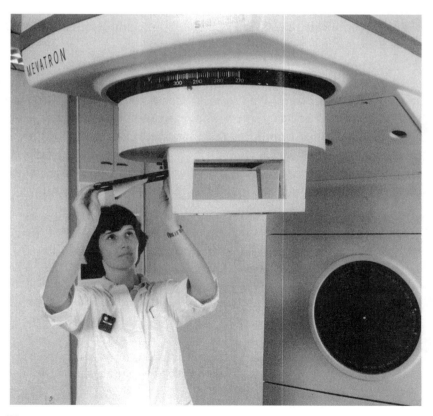

PEDIATRIC PATIENT SIMULATION

Simulation performed on children sometimes requires anesthesia, depending upon the ability of the child to cooperate. The same principles of immobilization for adults apply to pediatric patients. In most cases, an alphacradle is constructed for immobilization. In some situations, an aquaplast mask is necessary. A Velcro papoose can be used as a gentle restraint if the child is not sedated.

Treatment position depends on the body site being treated. For example, four-year-old Judy was treated for medulloblastoma, a malignant brain tumor in the **craniospinal axis** (brain and spinal cord). Judy was placed on her stomach. (See Figure 6-9.) Both an aquaplast mask and alphacradle were useful in her situation. Judy did not require sedation; we told her to pretend that she was traveling in a space ship.

For many types of treatments of the brain, children are placed on their backs. An aquaplast mask is used, almost always with an alphacradle for immobilization and for duplication of the same position each day of treatment. Placement on the back and the use of an alphacradle is common in treating abdominal, pelvic, and extremity malignancies as well.

Facing Page: Fig. 6-8. The technologist is sliding a blocking tray into the collimator. (Photo © 2002 by Siemens Medical Solutions. All rights reserved. Used with permission.)

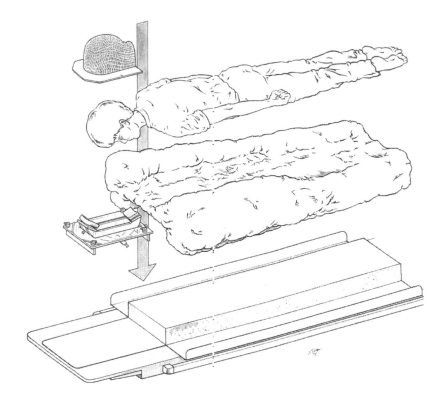

Fig. 6-9. Construction of an immobilization system for radiation therapy of the craniospinal axis. (Cranial Spinal Axis System by MED-TEC, Inc.Photo © 2001 by MED-TEC, Inc. All rights reserved. Used with permission.)

*"I try to avoid looking forward or backward,
and try to keep looking upward."*
– Charlotte Bronte

CHAPTER 7

WHAT TO EXPECT DURING AND AFTER RADIATION THERAPY

SIDE EFFECTS AND COMPLICATIONS FROM RADIATION THERAPY

In this chapter I describe the different body sites and the various site-specific side effects that might occur during radiation therapy. I also discuss measures that I take to minimize side effects. Additionally, I give examples of treatment positions, duration of treatment, and other important issues that my patients encounter.

Side effects fall into two categories, early (or **acute)**, and late (or **chronic)**. Acute side effects occur during or immediately after the course of treatment. Chronic side effects occur months or years later. Acute side effects are fairly common and are temporary. Chronic side effects are uncommon and can also be permanent; they are rarely serious.

Side effects from radiation therapy depend upon the body site that is being treated. This is in contrast to chemotherapy, a systemic treatment that travels throughout the body.

For example, if radiation therapy is prescribed to a patient's pelvis, it's possible that diarrhea or a change in the patient's urinary pattern will occur. On the other hand, if the patient receives radiation therapy to the chest for lung cancer, diarrhea is not an anticipated complication because there is no small intestine in the radiation therapy field.

Similarly, if treatment involves the neck area, nausea, vomiting, and diarrhea should not occur because the patient's stomach is not in the irradiated field. If the breast is treated, the patient might experience discoloration, peeling, darkening, and possibly burning of the skin of the breast. If the head is being treated, the patient can expect to lose some or all of her or his hair, depending on the amount of scalp included in the field.

Joanna, a 58-year-old math professor at the local university, was concerned that she would go bald while receiving radiation therapy to her pelvis for cancer of the endometrium. She was relieved to learn that this would not be the case.

A commonly reported symptom during the course of radiation therapy is fatigue. Patients are able to do everything they normally do, but they might feel more tired. (A discussion about fatigue appears in Chapter 10.)

When patients receive chemotherapy just before undergoing radiation therapy or at the same time, I make it a point to check their blood counts at least every other week. Should their white blood count, red blood count, or platelet count drop significantly, I need to make a decision about withholding radiation therapy and/or chemotherapy until the blood counts return to an acceptable level. Such interruption is usually no longer than two weeks. When necessary, I prescribe medications that stimulate the recovery of blood counts.

I advise all patients to practice birth control during the course of radiation therapy, regardless of which body site I am treating, as radiation therapy can cause a pregnant woman to have a miscarriage and can increase the risk of birth defects. In men, radiation therapy can lead to the production of abnormal sperm both during the treatment and for some time afterward.

Therefore, although there is no standard length of time that male and female patients should wait after radiation therapy concludes before attempting to conceive a child, I recommend that patients wait at least one year.

One of the most serious and rare late side effects from radiation therapy is radiation therapy-induced malignancy. Such second cancers, by definition, share three factors in common: they occur after the five-year anniversary of the completion of radiation therapy, they are a different cancer type than the original tumor, and they are within the radiation therapy field.

When we think of cancer statistics that are linked to nuclear blasts, such as Hiroshima and Chernobyl, we must make the distinction between nuclear fallout and cleanly prescribed radiation therapy. Although radiation therapy-induced malignancy can result from radiation therapy that was prescribed to treat any body site, its overall occurrence, fortunately, is less than five percent.

SIDE EFFECTS AND COMPLICATIONS FOR SPECIFIC BODY SITES

RADIATION THERAPY TO THE HEAD

Radiation therapy to the head area is used for a variety of malignant and benign conditions. Among some of the more commonly treated entities are: tumors of the brain; lesions of the orbits (bony sockets where the eyeballs are located); tumors of the pituitary gland; skin tumors of the scalp; and skin lesions of the face area. The number of treatments required depends on the type of tumor; it's something I tell my patients at the time of their consult.

Garrett, introduced in Chapter 6, needed 3-D conformal radiation therapy to his head for a malignant brain tumor. He required 33 treatments over seven weeks. I explained to Garrett that he should anticipate radiation-induced hair loss, usually after the third week of radiation therapy. The amount of hair that Garrett would lose depended on the volume of his scalp that was being irradiated. I informed Garrett that headaches, nausea, and vomiting are possible but unlikely side effects during the course of head radiation therapy. If these symptoms were to occur, steroids would be extremely helpful.

Bridgette, a 47-year-old breast cancer survivor, began radiation therapy to her left breast after she received chemotherapy. Chemotherapy caused Bridgette to lose her scalp hair, eyebrows, and eyelashes. These grew in again during the course of her radiation therapy, as these areas were not included in Bridgette's radiation therapy fields. Had she been treated with a field that encompassed her head, the radiation would have prevented hair regrowth at that time.

Philip, a 79-year-old retired commodities trader who had lung cancer, required whole brain radiation therapy for metastatic lesions to his brain. He received 15 treatments over three weeks. Because Philip's entire brain was being irradiated, he could expect to lose all his scalp hair — unlike Garrett, who was having only a segment of his brain treated and was anticipating only partial hair loss within the treated area. Because Garrett received treatment to one side of his head, he lost less hair on the other side. Philip also experienced some dryness of his scalp and along the tops and backs of his ears, which was easily treated with skin care products that I prescribed.

Radiation treatment for scalp tumors is similarly expected to produce only partial hair loss, again depending upon the volume of the scalp that is being irradiated. This was the case for Patricia, the 83-year-old woman introduced in Chapter 6 (in the section on skin lesions). For the skin cancer on the left side of her scalp, she received 15 treatments over three weeks. Patricia lost only the patch of hair that was within the radiation field.

Louise, a 58-year-old telephone operator, underwent 28 sessions over five and a half weeks to irradiate a benign tumor of the pituitary gland. She sustained some thinning of hair in the sideburn area, but no cosmetic defect.

Cynthia, a 54-year-old travel agent, underwent radiation therapy to the orbits (eye sockets) for benign thyroid-related eye disease. Cynthia underwent ten treatments over two weeks and experienced no hair loss.

To minimize the trauma of complete hair loss, I advise patients, especially women, to gradually shorten their hair over the first two weeks of radiation therapy. When the hair begins to thin, it can be removed entirely. The voluntary removal of hair is not only less devastating than letting it shed but also more hygienic.

As needed, I write prescriptions for a **cranial prosthesis**, or wig, the cost of which is reimbursed by many insurance companies. Patricia was able to cover up her partial hair loss with her overlying hair. She could have also used a partial hairpiece rather than a full wig.

Hair loss may be temporary or permanent, depending upon the dose of radiation. Therefore, hair loss associated with the dosage prescribed for brain metastases and for primary brain tumors is usually, but not always, permanent. Philip and Garrett had permanent hair loss. However, Patricia's hair grew back one year after her therapy.

Infrequently, if the middle ear has been included in the radiation therapy field, middle ear fluid can build up. Out of the hundreds of patients who had their middle ears included in the radiation fields, I am aware of only two who developed the full-blown problem. This complication was managed with the insertion of tubes, like those used in children, to evacuate fluid from the middle ear. In several other patients, this problem was not severe, and it was managed with antihistamine or decongestant medication.

When a patient undergoes whole brain radiation therapy, there is always the risk of long-term cognitive impairment — meaning difficulty with concentration, memory, organization, mathematics, learning, and other mental tasks. This complication is most commonly reported in children who have been treated with prophylactic, or preventive, brain radiation therapy for acute lymphocytic leukemia. It is less common in adults who have undergone brain irradiation to prevent the cells of small cell lung cancer that metastasized to the brain from growing into tumor masses. I am not aware of any patients whom I have treated who experienced cognitive impairments.

When children need to undergo radiation therapy to the brain, I routinely send the child for IQ testing beforehand to establish a baseline IQ. I would much rather see a child live with some degree of a learning impairment and receive remedial help in school than refuse treatment and never live to see a milestone such as graduation. Cognitive impairment is rare when **subtotal brain irradiation** is used, meaning that the radiation therapy field includes less than the whole brain. (In Chapter 4, in the section on physical and mental function, cognitive impairment is discussed in greater depth.)

Scattered radiation therapy to the lenses of the eyes can cause cataracts. Such a problem can be corrected surgically with cataract removal and the implantation of artificial lenses into one or both of the eyes. I am not aware of any of my patients sustaining radiation-induced cataracts.

When electron beam therapy is used to treat a lesion in or near the facial area, my staff of therapists places lead shields over the patient's eyelids to minimize the amount of scattered radiation to the lenses. For lesions located on the eyelid, therapists instill anesthetic eye drops and then insert a special lead contact lens into the affected eye before each treatment. (Refer to Figure 7-1 to see a picture of the eye shields. The contact lenses have a similar appearance.)

Whole brain radiation therapy or radiation therapy to the pituitary gland can be associated with diminished production of hormones by the pituitary gland. Such a complication can be corrected with hormone replacement medication. I send patients to an **endocrinologist**, a physician who specializes in diagnosing and correcting hormonal aberrations.

Be sure to discuss with your radiation oncologist whether you can drive safely, because some brain lesions can cause seizures, and you certainly don't want to experience a seizure while operating an automobile. (See the section entitled "Transportation Issues" in Chapter 4.)

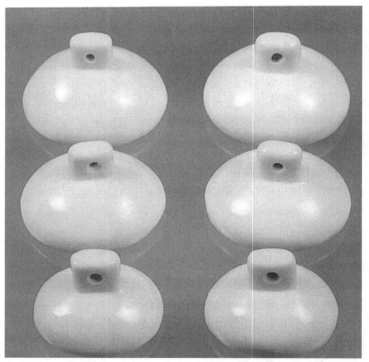

Fig. 7-1. Eye shields are placed over the patient's closed eyelids for daily treatment. They protect the eyes from scattered radiation. (Tungsten Eye Shields, MED-TEC, Inc.Photo © 2001 by MED-TEC, Inc. All rights reserved. Used with permission.)

RADIATION THERAPY TO THE HEAD AND NECK AREA

Radiation therapy to the head and neck area is used to treat tumors of the mouth, throat, larynx (voice box), nasopharynx (an air passage located behind the nose and above the top of mouth), nose, sinuses (air passages located behind the nose and above the roof of the mouth), salivary glands, the thyroid gland, and the neck. (See Figure 7-2 for a picture of head and neck anatomy.)

Jerry, a 59-year-old police officer, underwent surgery to remove a malignant tumor from his right tonsil. He required 30 radiation treatments over six weeks to his head and neck area. I advised Jerry that during the course of radiation therapy, it would be helpful to him to rinse his mouth and gargle with salt and soda washes. This mixture is made by adding one tablespoon of baking soda and one tablespoon of salt to a quart of water at room temperature. Jerry used this rinse as many times per day as he wished, and he found it quite cleansing and refreshing for both his mouth and throat. I told Jerry to avoid swallowing the solution, as the sodium load could cause his system to retain fluid.

Jerry found that room-temperature chamomile tea was also soothing. I advise avoiding commercial mouthwashes, however, because the chemical content can irritate the membranes that line the mouth and throat.

After Jerry's second week of radiation therapy, he experienced a sore throat and noticed ulcers in his mouth. I prescribed dietary modifications and medication to alleviate Jerry's discomfort. It was not necessary to stop radiation therapy because of these side effects.

Around the same period of time, Jerry noticed that his sense of taste was impaired. Food started to taste like cardboard. I advised him to use his sense of smell when he ate to help compensate for his diminished sense of taste.

Also at this time, Jerry noted dryness of his mouth. Unfortunately, this side effect was permanent. To help minimize his mouth dryness, I prescribed medication from the outset of Jerry's treatment that stimulated the flow of saliva. Jerry's mouth dryness would have been more severe had he not used the medication from the outset. I counseled him after he reported dryness to carry a water bottle at all times and to keep a flask of water at his bedside, so he might continually wet his mouth. When eating, he needed to drink copious amounts of liquid. In addition, to facilitate chewing and swallowing during meals, he found it helpful to moisturize his food with gravy.

Anatomy of the Head, Neck, Chest and Upper Abdomen

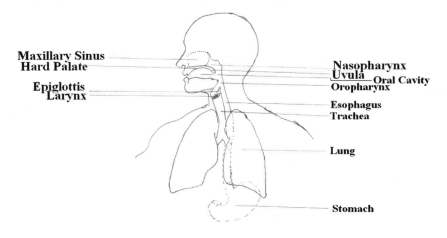

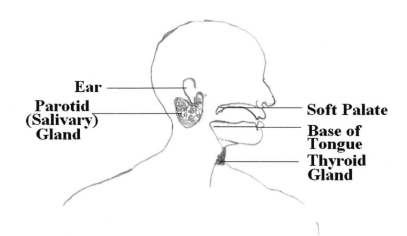

Fig. 7-2. Anatomy of the head, neck, chest, and upper abdomen. (Drawing courtesy of Danielle Feinstein. © 2002. All rights reserved. Used with permission.)

Jerry was instructed to brush and floss his teeth after each meal during the course of radiation therapy and to continue thereafter, throughout his lifetime. He was told to procure a travel toothbrush to have available when he ate away from home. The reason for the extra hygiene is that the dry mouth caused by radiation therapy also caused changes in the chemical composition of his saliva. The normal bacteria that live in the mouth change as the pH of the saliva changes, putting Jerry at substantial risk for cavities and other dental complications. Brushing and flossing after every meal minimizes these complications, and might even prevent them altogether.

Before radiation therapy begins, it is my policy to send all patients who have any of their natural teeth to the dentist. I ask the dentist to do a thorough cleaning at that time. Additionally, I request that impressions be taken of the patient's natural teeth so that **fluoride gel carrier trays** might be constructed. These trays look like the kind of mouth guards that athletes wear.

In Jerry's case, he placed fluoride gel inside his carrier trays. He wore the trays on his teeth for approximately ten minutes every day, finding that he was able to do this while reading the newspaper, watching TV, or otherwise relaxing. The extra coating of fluoride did wonders to protect Jerry's teeth from decaying. Because dry mouth is permanent and Jerry's teeth were always at risk for breakdown, his use of the fluoride gel carriers needed to be continued throughout his lifetime, not stopping when radiation therapy was finished. I made Jerry aware that if he were to develop a dental infection that required dental extraction (the pulling of a tooth), he could experience serious injury to his jawbone — an example of an ounce of prevention being worth a pound of cure.

Patients who wear full or partial dentures might need to refrain from wearing them during radiation therapy to the head and neck area, as dentures might be irritating. Thus, Jerry did not wear his partial dentures during the period of time he was receiving radiation therapy. I told him that new dentures should not be made for several months following the therapy, because the jawbones tend to undergo changes, known as remodeling, as a result of radiation. Until the remodeling process stabilized, new dentures would not fit properly. Ultimately, he had new partial dentures constructed one year after he completed radiation therapy.

In addition, I prescribed **range of motion exercises** for Jerry. The **temporomandibular joint**, commonly called **TMJ**, is the joint that controls the opening and closing of the mouth. I made Jerry aware that if he were to develop scar tissue in the joint, it might restrict the range of motion of his lower jaw — the ability to open his mouth fully. By practicing these exercises, Jerry minimized such a complication.

I also prescribed exercises for Jerry to limit his losing the range of motion of his neck. Radiation therapy can cause what is called woody fibrosis, or scarring of the neck muscles. This complication is more common in patients who have undergone neck dissection(s), surgery to remove the lymph nodes of the neck. Such scarring can limit the range of motion of neck muscles, but preventive or prophylactic exercises can minimize long-term difficulty. Jerry lost none of his range of motion.

He did, however, experience temporary hoarseness during the course of his radiation therapy. Therefore, it became important for him to minimize talking and whispering, and to rely more on the use of body language and writing to communicate. His hoarseness resolved four weeks after he completed radiation therapy.

He also found that his skin in the treated area temporarily became red and dry. This included the skin behind his ears and on his earlobes, face, and neck. In addition, he experienced mild cracking of the skin of his neck and his earlobes, for which I prescribed skin care products. Jerry lost some of the beard within the irradiated areas of his face and neck, though he didn't mind.

I informed Jerry that during the course of radiation therapy to the head and neck, it is desirable not to let radiation-induced side effects interrupt treatment. Instead, he'd be given medication and other supportive measures to minimize the severity of such side effects. The exception would be if he had a severe skin reaction; namely, a burn. In such an instance, it is necessary to hold treatment and allow the skin to heal before resuming radiation therapy. Medication would also be applied to the burn to expedite skin healing.

Theresa, a 78-year-old former restaurant owner, had a malignant tumor of her left vocal cord, which is part of the larynx. She did not require radiation therapy to the whole neck because it is rare to have lymph node metastases (the spread of cancer to the lymph nodes) result from a vocal cord tumor. Although Theresa received 28 treatments over five and a half weeks, the small field being treated spared Theresa from most of the side effects that Jerry incurred, except for hoarseness and sore throat.

Both Jerry's and Theresa's treatment fields included the thyroid gland, putting its function at risk for becoming impaired in the future. If they developed **hypothyroidism**, meaning that if their thyroids had become underactive, they would have received medication to replace the hormone that the thyroid gland was no longer producing adequately.

After lymph nodes of the neck have been surgically removed and radiation has taken place, it is common for patients to develop a fat pad under the chin called a dewlap. This side effect is chronic, and in Jerry's case it became noticeable several months after his radiation treatments ended. He found it necessary to wear a larger collar size because of the dewlap.

I explained to Jerry that if the dosage of radiation to the spinal cord were to exceed what we identify as **tolerance** — the maximum dosage that the spinal cord can receive before it becomes damaged — he could become paraplegic or quadriplegic. He was pleased to learn that in the modern radiation therapy era, such a complication is virtually unheard of.

Jerry was apprised of the fact that patients who've received radiation therapy to the head and neck area occasionally report feeling a sensation like an electric shock in their spine and tingling or pain in their hands when they flex their necks forward. This is not a serious problem but rather a mild annoyance. Its medical name is **L'Hermitte's sign**. If this side effect were to occur, Jerry might not notice it until several months after radiation therapy ended. L'Hermitte's sign resolves by itself after several more months.

CHEST (THORACIC) RADIATION THERAPY

Inga, (described in Chapter 6 in the section on chest simulation), required 25 treatments over five weeks, along with chemotherapy, for cancer of the esophagus. Livia, whose case was presented in the same section of Chapter 6, needed 36 fractions (or daily treatments) over seven weeks for lung cancer, also with chemotherapy.

Both of these women were counseled that the skin within the radiation therapy field might become red, dry, dark, or sensitive. If that were to happen, I would prescribe skin care products.

Because the esophagus was included in Inga's and Livia's radiation therapy fields, I explained to each the risk of esophagitis — inflammation of the esophagus. The esophagus is the tube that connects the mouth to the stomach, traveling through the chest. Esophagitis would feel as if the patient were swallowing broken glass or sandpaper. I made it clear to Inga and Livia that esophagitis would be temporary and could be managed with dietary modifications and medications. Both women were aware that esophagitis was a strong possibility because it usually occurs in patients who are receiving concurrent radiation therapy and chemotherapy. Inga noticed she'd developed esophagitis during the third week of radiation therapy. Livia did not develop it, however.

Inga and Livia were advised that if they noticed any change in their usual coughs during or shortly after their courses of radiation therapy, they would need to report it to me. **Radiation pneumonitis** is a form of pneumonia induced by radiation therapy. It is self-limited; that is, if nothing is done, it resolves by itself. However, I usually prescribe cough syrup and Prednisone (Roxane & Watson Laboratories, Inc.), a steroid. Together they speed the healing process.

Chronic or late complications are much less common. I discussed with Inga and Livia the possibility of **radiation-induced lung fibrosis**, which means that scar tissue could be produced in the areas of the lung that were within the radiation therapy portals, or fields. To be thorough, before Livia began radiation therapy, I sent her for pulmonary function tests that assessed her breathing. Inga's radiation fields included a minuscule volume of lung, so she did not require pulmonary function tests. If Livia's tests indicated that she had poor lung reserve, I would have needed to compromise on the size of the radiation therapy field. Fortunately, this was not the case. I counseled Livia that if she were to develop radiation-induced lung fibrosis, it probably would not cause any consequence such as worsening of her breathing; rather, it was likely to be noticed on a CAT scan months or years later.

Livia and Inga were each advised of the possibility that they could develop an **esophageal stricture**, meaning a leathery-textured, scarred, narrowing of the esophagus. If this were to happen, the stricture would be managed by **dilation**, a procedure that stretches the esophagus back to an appropriate diameter.

Each patient was also told that injury to the spinal cord was exceedingly rare. With properly performed radiation therapy, most likely there would be no complications related to the spinal cord.

Bernard, a 55-year-old letter carrier, required post-operative radiation therapy to his chest for a malignant tumor of his thymus gland. He received 25 treatments over five weeks. I made him aware of the same potential complications. In addition, I told Bernard there might be a thinning of the chest hair within the radiation therapy portals. In the end, Bernard had slight thinning of his chest hair, but it was not at all bothersome to him.

RADIATION THERAPY TO THE ABDOMEN

Abdominal radiation therapy is used to treat tumors of the stomach, intestines, testicles, kidneys, adrenal glands, ovaries, and pancreas. Richard, introduced in Chapter 6 (in the section on abdominal simulation), required post-operative radiation therapy for stomach cancer. He required 25 treatments over five weeks. Because Richard's stomach was in the radiation therapy field, I anticipated that during the course of his radiation therapy he might experience nausea and vomiting. Fortunately, a great deal of medication was available to minimize Richard's nausea, and it prevented him from vomiting, as well.

Richard was cautioned that he might develop abdominal cramping and diarrhea during the course of radiation therapy, because loops of intestine were within the radiation therapy fields. Richard was told to procure over-the-counter anti-diarrhea medication. If necessary, I would have prescribed another medication for cramping. I told Richard that if these measures failed to control diarrhea, his treatment would have been put on hold for several days until his diarrhea resolved, after which he would have resumed radiation therapy safely. Fortunately, Richard had only mild diarrhea that was controlled by diet and over-the-counter medication. He required no interruption of his treatment course.

I made Richard aware of the less-common side effects that could occur months or years later, such as possible injury to loops of intestine, resulting in malabsorption syndrome. If the latter were to occur, he would need to take medication to supplement the digestive enzymes that his intestines normally produced. Richard was similarly advised that fewer than five percent of patients incur severe damage to the intestine requiring an operation to remove the portion of the damaged intestine.

Richard's stomach area lay in close proximity to his kidneys. It was inevitable that segments of both kidneys would be included in the radiation therapy field. These segments of kidneys were at risk for becoming nonfunctional months later. Fortunately, the portions of the kidneys that were not irradiated would compensate. I was extremely careful to exclude as much kidney as possible. Richard's kidney function blood tests have remained normal to the present, nearly one year since the period of radiation therapy ended.

Also located in the vicinity of Richard's stomach is his liver. Thus, part of it was inevitably included in the treatment field. I informed Richard that months or years later, that section of liver might become nonfunctional. However, the remainder of the liver that was excluded from the treatment field would function normally and compensate for the damaged segment of liver. His liver function blood tests have also remained normal.

I informed Richard that if the radiation therapy dose to his spinal cord were to exceed tolerance — the maximum dose that the spinal cord could receive before becoming damaged — he could become quadriplegic or paraplegic. However, I reassured him that in the era of modern radiation therapy, such a complication is virtually unheard of.

RADIATION THERAPY TO THE PELVIS

Pelvic radiation therapy is used to treat tumors of gynecologic origin (such as the cervix, vagina, uterus, and ovaries), cancer of the bladder, rectal cancer, anal cancer, prostate cancer, testicular cancer, lymphomas, and miscellaneous conditions.

Doris, (whose case was presented in Chapter 6 in the section on pelvic simulation), required pelvic radiation therapy for rectal cancer. She received 30 treatments over six weeks.

Doris was made aware that diarrhea and abdominal cramping are common side effects during the course of her type of radiation therapy, and that I would take every measure to limit the amount of small intestine included in her radiation therapy fields. The less intestine in the field, the lower the rate of diarrhea.

Because Doris had no problem retaining a full bladder of urine, I advised her to drink as much liquid as she could a half-hour before her daily treatments. Her outstretched bladder displaced loops of small intestine up and out of her pelvis. She therefore had no diarrhea or cramping. If she had, I would have managed her symptoms with medication and dietary modification. Interrupting the course of radiation therapy because of diarrhea was unlikely.

I also made Doris aware of other possible side effects. I said she might experience burning upon urination, frequency of urination, and other symptoms that mimic a urinary tract infection. If that occurred, I would prescribe medication to reduce these side effects. However, if I suspected that she had an actual urinary tract infection, she would have been asked to submit a sample of urine to confirm or refute this possibility. If an infection had been confirmed, I would have prescribed appropriate antibiotics.

I described to Doris the possibility of irritation of the skin between her buttocks or in the area of the groin. If such a reaction were to occur, it would not usually warrant interruption of the course of radiation therapy and would be treated with skin care products. Also, on learning that it is not uncommon for the pubic hair to become more sparse or lost, Doris wasn't fazed about the possibility of such a side effect.

I explained that she might feel vaginal irritation and dryness during the course of her radiation therapy. Irritation would be managed with vinegar and water vaginal douches; vaginal lubricants and moisturizers would be helpful during intercourse.

I informed her of the possibility that her vagina might become tender and narrowed, and that after completing radiation therapy she would be given a vaginal dilator to use at home several times a week. (Please refer to the section on sexuality in Chapter 4.)

Doris completed radiation therapy two years ago. She continues to use her dilator several times a week when she lies in bed, leaving it in place for approximately ten minutes while she watches TV or listens to the radio. After using the dilator, she washes it with soap and water.

Before her radiation treatment began, Doris was post-menopausal. Women who are pre-menopausal usually become menopausal secondary to pelvic radiation therapy. I advise menstruating women to be monitored for signs of menopause, so that decisions about hormone replacement therapy can be made.

Doris' rectum and anus were removed at the time of her operation. Patients who have not had this type of surgery occasionally report burning inside the rectum after the second week of radiation therapy. In such cases, I prescribe a medicated suppository to relieve the inflammation.

For patients who experience burning in the anal area because of frequent wiping or from a radiation-induced burn, **Sitz baths** are very helpful. The patient places the Sitz bath on his or her toilet and fills it with warm water. It soothes the skin of the anal area. I prescribe anal skin care products, as well.

Doris was counseled that long-term side effects from radiation therapy are much less common than short-term side effects. Nevertheless, it was possible for her to have damage to her large intestine. This injury could manifest itself as chronic mucus and bloody discharge from the surgically reconstructed bowel. Such a problem would usually be managed with medication or laser surgery. If there were severe damage to the small or large intestine, surgery might be necessary to remove the damaged portion of bowel. Yet, this complication is rare. Even more rarely, patients who have not had a previous colostomy might need one. Fortunately, such a severe complication occurs in fewer than five percent of patients. Doris had no long-term bowel complications.

Similarly, if there were severe damage to her bladder, Doris was told that it might be necessary to have her bladder surgically removed and to wear a bag on the side of her abdomen to collect urine. Again, this complication is exceedingly rare. More common, but still very infrequent, are persistent irritable bladder symptoms such as urinary frequency, burning, and weak stream, but these are readily managed with medication.

Vincent (whom I introduced in Chapter 2 and again in Chapter 6 in the section on pelvic simulation) was treated for prostate cancer with 3-D conformal radiation therapy. Six fields were used to treat his prostate. He required 40 treatments over eight weeks. If a prostate seed implant had been a component of his radiation therapy, Vincent would have required 25 treatments over five weeks. The field sizes were relatively small. Most of the normal, surrounding bladder and rectum were excluded from the irradiated fields.

To anticipate any acute complications, I discussed with Vincent the possibility that the small field sizes would likely limit the side effects to urinary burning, frequent urination, weak stream, diarrhea, and rectal burning. Potential late complications that he faced included rectal damage and bladder damage, as I describe above in relation to Doris's potential. Again, however, such late complications are rare.

Vincent was told that impotence and loss of libido have been reported after pelvic radiation therapy, but are more common after patients have undergone major pelvic surgery for cancer. Vincent did not have surgery. Impotence is a common side effect from hormonal agents, which in Vincent's case he'd been taking before his radiation therapy. I advised him that incontinence of stool and urine has been reported but is more common following a major cancer operation.

It was possible for Vincent to develop a **urethral stricture**, meaning that the tube that drains urine from his bladder to his penis could become scarred and narrowed. It could take months or even years for a urethral stricture to form, and if it did, Vincent might have to undergo dilation, or stretching, of the stricture so that the tube could return to an appropriate diameter. Again, this is an extremely uncommon complication.

For Pedro, (the six-year-old boy with leukemia whom I introduced in Chapter 6 in the section on pelvic simulation), I told his parents that when the testicles are irradiated, skin reaction is possible, but unlikely. (Please see the section about radiation therapy to the skin in this chapter.)

Infertility for both males and females becomes an issue any time the pelvis is treated. The total dose of radiation that the ovaries or testes receive determines whether fertility will be preserved or lost. Patients for whom future childbearing is desired need to be counseled about sperm or egg banking.

RADIATION THERAPY TO THE SKIN

Skin radiation therapy is used for a variety of malignancies and for some benign skin disorders. The most commonly treated entities include basal cell carcinoma, squamous cell carcinoma, Kaposi's sarcoma, and lymphomas of the skin. Occasionally, melanomas are treated with primary radiation therapy instead of surgery.

Wilbur, the 82-year-old retired liquor store owner, (discussed in Chapter 6 in the section on skin lesion simulation), had a small lesion and therefore required 15 treatments over three weeks. Peggy, the 85-year-old retired clerk introduced just before Wilbur, had a larger cancer on her nose. She required 35 treatments over seven weeks.

Peggy and Wilbur were individually counseled that acute side effects are confined to the irradiated area and usually include redness of the skin, sunburn sensation, darkening of the skin, peeling, itching, drying, blistering, and third degree burning. The severity of side effects depends upon the dose and the size of the field. It makes sense that Peggy's acute skin reaction was more intense than Wilbur's. I prescribed a skin care product for both Wilbur and Peggy when they began radiation treatment to minimize skin reaction and to help treat skin reactions when they occurred.

The x-rays of the linear accelerator deliver a minimal dose to the skin. This dose builds to its maximum at a fraction of an inch below the skin surface. The electron beam gives a much more significant dose to the skin, but it, too, achieves its maximum dose beneath the surface of the skin. When the external beam radiation dose needs to treat the surface of the skin, such as when treating skin cancer or the chest wall after a mastectomy has been performed, bolus material is placed in the treatment field, as I discussed in Chapter 6. Bolus material was placed on both Peggy's and Wilbur's lesions for each treatment. (See Figure 6-6 for a photo of bolus material.)

For Peggy, after the fourth week of treatment, it was necessary to suspend radiation therapy for several days until her skin burn healed. If either patient had experienced pain related to the skin reaction, I would have also prescribed appropriate pain medication.

When Peggy's facial skin lesion was treated, her eyes and nostrils were protected. (See Figure 7-1 for a picture of eye shields.) These devices block scattered radiation from penetrating the lens of the eye and from the lining of the nostril, respectively.

When patients have skin cancers that are on or near the lips, smooth lead strips are inserted between the inner aspect of the lip and the gums before each treatment to minimize ulceration inside the mouth.

Peggy and Wilbur were told that it would be beneficial to apply moisturizing cream to the irradiated skin daily throughout their lifetimes. They were also told that months or years later, the irradiated skin might be either paler or darker than it was originally. Most patients find this an acceptable cosmetic outcome.

Peggy and Wilbur were also informed that thin, threadlike blood vessels, called **telangiectases**, could start to show through the skin in the irradiated area months or years after treatment. These seldom pose any significant cosmetic deformity. As it turned out, Wilbur had mild darkening of his irradiated skin and Peggy had a few telangiectases. Both patients were happy with their cosmetic outcomes.

Wilbur was told that any hair within the irradiated field on his back might be lost, temporarily or permanently. Wilbur was not concerned. (Please refer to the section regarding hair loss at the end of Chapter 4, in the section on cosmetic appearance.)

RADIATION THERAPY TO THE BREAST AND CHEST WALL

Liz, introduced in Chapter 6 (in the section on breast and chest wall simulation), required right breast radiation therapy after a right lumpectomy had been performed. Genevieve, introduced in the same section, required adjuvant radiation therapy to her left chest wall because she had high-risk features for chest wall recurrence after her mastectomy. In my practice, I also prescribe chest wall radiation therapy for patients who have had nodules on the chest wall secondary to recurrent breast cancer.

In Genevieve's case, I decided it was necessary to irradiate lymph nodes in her supraclavicular area (lower neck) and in her axilla (underarm area), based upon information from the **pathology report** of her primary breast cancer and axillary lymph nodes.

Liz required 28 treatments to her right breast over five and a half weeks and Genevieve needed 28 treatments to her left chest wall, also over five and a half weeks. Breast and chest wall radiation treatment typically entails 28 treatments to the entire breast or chest wall, followed by a boost or cone down to the lumpectomy bed or to the mastectomy scar for an additional five treatments over one week. The total number of treatments is 33 over a period of six and a half weeks. Bolus material was used on Genevieve's chest wall field and mastectomy scar cone down.

The lymph nodes of Genevieve's lower neck and underarm required fewer treatments than her chest wall, and all areas were treated concurrently.

Patients who undergo lumpectomy, but who have a significant number of axillary lymph nodes that test positive for cancer cells, require radiation therapy not only to the breast but also to the supraclavicular fossa and possibly to the underarm.

The most difficult part of the irradiation process for both Liz and Genevieve was having to lie on the firm table with an arm extended up and over their heads, supported by the breast board. For each woman, the extended arm was the one on the side being treated, whereas her head was kept turned to the opposite side.

Because Genevieve received chemotherapy and was irradiated with bolus on her chest wall, her skin reaction was more pronounced than Liz's. (Please see the section about skin reaction in this chapter.) Skin reactions are also more common in women with large breasts who have a prominent fold under the breast. The most common areas to burn or blister are the areas under the crease of the breast and under the arm. I told Liz and Genevieve that it was ideal for them to go braless. Because this was not practical for Liz, her best choice was a cotton bra without an underwire. I recommended a sports bra that fit below the crease of the breast.

Genevieve was told that skin reactions were unavoidable as a result of irradiating her chest wall. Once radiation therapy began, I gave Liz and Genevieve moisturizing skin cream to apply, which helped to minimize their skin reaction. Genevieve developed burns, so I gave her additional instructions. Once her skin reaction settled down, it was reasonable for her to continue to apply the moisturizer to the irradiated skin daily to minimize dryness.

Treatment to Genevieve's chest wall needed to be suspended for a week until the burn healed. Liz proceeded through treatment without interruption. Had she experienced a burn, I would have proceeded to treat her cone down to the lumpectomy bed, as long as the burn was not within the cone down site. In this way, provided that the burn resolved, no time would be lost and the treatment of the breast fields would resume after her five cone down treatments were completed.

Because the lymph nodes in Genevieve's lower neck were being included in the treatment field, she was advised of the possibility of developing a sore throat during the course of radiation therapy. This did occur after the third week of radiation therapy, so I prescribed appropriate measures. Radiation therapy to this field did not need to be put on hold, however, as her sore throat was tolerable.

As a result of irradiation to her lower neck and underarm, she also experienced a skin reaction on the back of her shoulder on the treated side. This occurred because the radiation therapy beam exited through her shoulder after being directed to the lymph nodes in the lower neck; in addition, radiation therapy to the underarm was delivered through the back of Genevieve's shoulder. Genevieve used the moisturizing cream to ease discomfort. Pain medication would have been prescribed if Genevieve had any discomfort, but luckily she had none.

Liz did not receive chemotherapy, and as no significant drops in her blood counts were anticipated, only a baseline blood count was needed. Liz was using Tamoxifen, which is also known as Nolvadex (Astra Zeneca Pharmaceuticals) and which usually does not affect a patient's blood counts. Genevieve, on the other hand, had recently completed a course of chemotherapy, so I ordered a blood count every other week.

Liz and Genevieve were told that at the end of their courses of radiation therapy, or shortly after, they might experience a dry cough or a change in their baseline cough. Occasionally, radiation therapy can cause a form of pneumonia called radiation pneumonitis. (Please refer to the discussion of radiation pneumonitis in the section entitled "Chest (Thoracic) Radiation Therapy" earlier in this chapter.)

Liz and Genevieve were each made aware of the possibility that months or years later, scar tissue could be produced in the sliver of lung that lies within the radiation therapy field. Since I took the necessary measures to limit the amount of lung in their radiation therapy fields, if scar tissue did develop, it would rarely be consequential; rather, it would be an incidental finding on an x-ray or CAT scan done for some other purpose.

Because Genevieve's left chest wall was irradiated, there was some risk of injury to her heart. Therefore, I took every precaution to minimize the amount of heart encompassed within the field. With careful CAT scan-guided planning, it is rare to experience complications to heart vessels, the outer lining of the heart, or the heart muscle.

Although radiation therapy to the breast and chest wall encompasses ribs, it is very rare to see fractures of the ribs. Nevertheless, both Liz and Genevieve were told about this risk. When the chest wall has been irradiated, it is not uncommon to see, months or years later, telangiectases develop on the chest wall. These usually do not cause any significant cosmetic deformity or symptoms.

When necessary to treat lymph nodes in the lower neck or the armpit, another possibility is **lymphedema**, or swelling of the arm. Lymphedema is unusual in patients who do not have axillary (underarm) lymph nodes removed. When only the lymph nodes in the lower neck are treated, the risk is not great. However, when it is necessary to include lymph nodes at the top of the underarm, the risk of arm swelling is nearly 40 percent. This is a permanent consequence that is unfortunately unsightly and uncomfortable.

I explained this risk carefully to Genevieve. If she had chosen to refuse radiation therapy to the underarm, I would have respected her decision. However, it was important for Genevieve to weigh the benefits and risks, because tumor recurrence in the underarm is also a major complication.

Irradiating Genevieve's lower neck raised the possibility, though rare, of another complication: **brachial plexopathy**. This is damage to the cluster of nerves located in the lower neck which affects sensation and arm movement on the side that is treated. Such damage could cause tingling in the arm or weakness of the arm.

An occasional patient may complain of shoulder stiffness before, during, or after radiation therapy. Usually this is noticed by patients who've had surgery to remove the lymph nodes of the underarm. Because Genevieve was affected, she practiced exercises that I prescribed before her simulation. If necessary, I would have requested a physical therapy consult, although she did not need physical therapy. The passage of time was all that was needed for Genevieve.

(Breast tenderness during and after radiation therapy is something I discuss in Chapter 4 in the section about sexuality after a cancer diagnosis.)

Another possibility is that over the course of time, the treated breast might retract and become shorter than it was after surgery. Although breast retraction happened to Liz, she felt that the cosmetic outcome was nevertheless quite good, and that preserving her breast was preferable to having a mastectomy followed by reconstruction.

Both Liz and Genevieve completed radiation therapy several years ago, and neither has had any adverse long-term side effects.

RADIATION THERAPY TO THE EXTREMITIES

Radiation therapy to the arms and legs is most commonly used for metastatic bone tumors (discussed later in this chapter). Less commonly, extremities are irradiated for sarcomas of soft tissue and for primary bone sarcomas.

In Mary's case, which I presented in Chapter 6 (in the section on simulation of the extremities), she received 33 treatments over six and a half weeks. I informed her that when the radiation therapy field must cross a joint, such as the elbow joint, it is possible for scar tissue to build up in the joint space months or years later. This complication could limit the range of motion of the affected joint. However, I let her know that physical therapy to minimize disability, and even to prevent such a complication, would be prescribed when radiation therapy began.

Mary's surgical scar was encompassed in the radiation therapy field, and bolus material was placed over it for daily treatments. A burn developed, but it healed after her radiation treatments were suspended for one week, during which time she used a skin care product. Please see the section in this chapter for a discussion of skin reactions.

IRRADIATION OF BONES

This type of radiation therapy is usually done for metastatic disease or for multiple myeloma to palliate pain and fractures. Occasionally, radiation therapy is used for primary bone sarcomas. Dave, (whose case I discussed in Chapter 6 in the section on bone simulation), received ten treatments to his ribs over two weeks.

I informed Dave that it is not common to sustain skin darkening, skin reddening, or hair loss within the radiation therapy portals. However, when ribs are treated with the electron beam, instead of x-rays, some reddening and darkening of the skin is more likely to occur. Other than a residual, faint darkening, any skin reaction is temporary and is managed with skin care products.

Clayton (introduced in Chapter 6 in the section on simulation of the extremities) received ten treatments to his hip joint over two weeks. I told Clayton that ulceration occasionally occurs in the crease of the groin.

When vertebral bodies or vertebrae (bones that make up the spine) are irradiated, side effects are dependent upon the body site that is treated. Ben (whose case I presented in Chapter 6 in the section on bone simulation) had his upper (cervical) spine treated. I told him that he might experience a sore throat, dry mouth, thickened saliva, and an altered sense of taste. (Also see the discussion earlier in this chapter on radiation therapy to the head and neck.) If the middle of Ben's spine (thoracic) had been irradiated, which it wasn't, he might have developed esophagitis. Please see the section earlier in this chapter on chest (thoracic) radiation therapy.

Dorothy (introduced in Chapter 6 in the section on bone simulation) was counseled about the possibility of developing abdominal cramping and diarrhea when her lower spine (lumbar and sacral) received treatment. (Please see the section earlier in this chapter on radiation therapy to the abdomen.)

RADIATION THERAPY FOR HODGKIN'S DISEASE

Radiation therapy for Hodgkin's disease is classically delivered through a field called a mantle field (described in Chapter 6.)

Matthew (whose case was presented in Chapter 6 beginning with the section on simulation of the mantle field) received 20 treatments over four weeks. Before initiating radiation therapy to the mantle field, I referred Matthew to his dentist. (To understand why dental evaluation is necessary, please see the section earlier in this chapter on radiation therapy to the head and neck area.) I carefully explained these side effects to him.

Matthew did not receive chemotherapy. In patients who do, especially when their regimen includes Prednisone, I taper off Prednisone very gradually during the course of radiation therapy. Such a precaution helps to minimize and prevent radiation pneumonitis. Please see the discussion on radiation pneumonitis earlier in this chapter in the section on chest (thoracic) radiation therapy.

The mantle field includes hair at the nape of neck. Hair loss in this area is usually temporary but might be permanent. Fortunately, the cosmetic result is reasonable because overlying hair can cover the radiation-induced hair loss. Loss of the lower part of the beard is also common and is usually temporary. Matthew did not have any cosmetic impairment.

Skin reaction was unlikely for Matthew but is more common for patients who receive radiation therapy after chemotherapy. The most common sites for a skin reaction are on the ear lobes, in the creases of the neck, and in the underarms. It is usually not necessary to interrupt radiation therapy for such a reaction. I prescribe skin cream to prevent and treat burns.

Matthew experienced queasiness because the upper aspect of his stomach projected into his mantle field. Dietary advice was given and antinausea medication prescribed. Matthew tolerated his treatments fairly well.

I carefully explained to him that side effects could occur months or years later, and although those would be less common, they could be more serious. The most common long-term side effect is hypothyroidism. (This side effect is discussed earlier in this chapter in the section on radiation therapy to the head and neck area.)

I educated Matthew about the need for preventive dental care and oral hygiene to be carried out throughout his lifetime, as he would always be at risk for dental decay and its secondary complications to the jawbone. By practicing preventive measures, he could see that such complications remained rare. I informed Matthew that dry mouth was not uncommon following mantle radiation therapy but was usually temporary. (Please see the section on radiation therapy to the head and neck earlier in this chapter to learn about measures to help relieve dry mouth.)

Radiation-induced heart disease has been reported in the literature. It is more common in patients who have received Adriamycin (Pharmacia & Upjohn Company). Side effects on the heart can affect the heart vessels, the muscles of the heart, and the sac that surrounds the heart. I told Matthew that he would be monitored over the years for such complications, and that if any abnormality were suspected, action would be taken to prevent any serious problems.

I told Matthew that permanent scarring of the segments of his lungs that were included in the radiation therapy fields was a possibility, but it would probably cause no consequences such as shortness of breath. It was more likely to be something noticed on a CAT scan that was obtained for some other reason.

It was discussed with Matthew that when radiation to both a mantle field and an abdominal lymph node/spleen field are prescribed, injury to the spinal cord is rare. With properly performed radiation therapy, there should be no complications related to the spinal cord.

It was necessary to treat the lymph nodes of Matthew's abdomen and his spleen. These areas comprise another classic radiation field used to treat Hodgkin's disease. Matthew received 17 treatments over three and a half weeks to this area.

I also talked with Matthew about the side effects associated with this treatment field: nausea and vomiting. Fortunately, medication that I prescribed minimized such side effects. Diarrhea was also possible but could be managed with medication and diet.

When the spleen is irradiated, patients are vulnerable to certain infections. Therefore, I prescribed specific vaccinations for Matthew to prevent particular infectious complications.

I told Matthew that shingles was one of the most common infectious complications that could occur during or after radiation therapy. I counseled him that if he were to notice any pain, itching, or rash he should make me aware. Medication exists that can limit the course of shingles and can expedite the healing process. Also, pain medication can be prescribed.

As I stated earlier in this chapter, one of the most serious late side effects from radiation therapy is radiation-induced malignancy. Although this complication can occur after radiation therapy has been used to treat any body site, its overall incidence is less than five percent. However, in Hodgkin's disease, the reported incidence of radiation-induced cancer is approximately ten percent.

Second malignancies induced by radiation therapy are more common in patients who receive both chemotherapy and radiation therapy. Patients who have been irradiated for Hodgkin's disease require careful follow-up throughout their lives. It is important to remember that the benefit of curing Hodgkin's disease is much greater than the risk of incurring a second malignancy. I reminded Matthew to focus on this benefit.

"Thou shall not worry,
for worry is the most unproductive
of all human activities."
— Author unknown

CHAPTER 8

SPECIAL FORMS OF RADIATION THERAPY

BRACHYTHERAPY

Brachytherapy is the term used to describe internal radiation therapy and radiation applied directly to the body surface. Brachytherapy can be used as a single radiation therapy modality, or its use might either predate or follow external beam radiation therapy. Your radiation oncologist will explain to you what is necessary to appropriately treat your tumor.

Brachytherapy can be used to deliver radiation therapy to nearly all body sites. The process delivers a very high dose of radiation therapy to intended sites and very little to the normal, surrounding tissue.

Radioactive materials called isotopes are applied to the localized tumor on the body surface or are introduced into cancerous tissue via an **insertion** or implant. Brachytherapy is either temporary or permanent.

Hollow metal or plastic applicators are inserted into body tissues and are then loaded with the brachytherapy source or sources. For temporary insertions and implants, the sources and their applicators are removed after the desired dose of radiation therapy has been delivered.

Intracavitary insertions are used to place the radioactive isotopes into body cavities such as the uterus and the vagina. Ruth, a 70-year-old tennis coach, underwent a hysterectomy for endometrial cancer. To reduce the risk of cancer recurrence in her vagina, a vaginal cylinder was inserted. (For a photo of a vaginal cylinder, see Figure 8-1.)

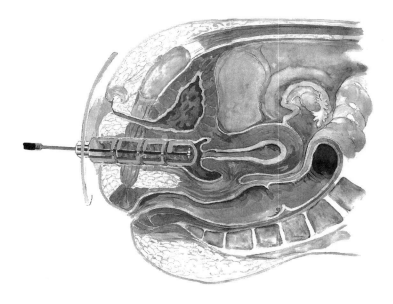

Fig. 8-1. A vaginal cylinder insertion for brachytherapy to the vagina. (Photo © 1995 by Nucletron Corporation. All rights reserved. Used with permission.)

Intraluminal insertions are introduced into body cavities such as the airways. Douglas, a 66-year-old construction worker, received the maximum dose of external beam radiation therapy to his chest for lung cancer. However, his tumor did not regress completely, and he continued to cough up blood. Therefore, he underwent a lung insertion, which succeeded in controlling his bleeding.

The term **interstitial brachytherapy** refers to an implant. The implant might be permanent or temporary. For example, in cases of prostate cancer, permanent sources of radioactive material, called seeds, are introduced into the prostate gland surgically. In cancers of the head and neck, temporary implants are introduced into tumors and are removed after the desired dose of radiation therapy has been delivered. Occasionally after a lumpectomy has been performed, a temporary breast implant is performed in lieu of an electron beam boost.

MAMMOSITE RADIATION THERAPY SYSTEM (RTS)

· The MammoSite Radiation Therapy System (RTS), made by Proxima Therapeutics, Inc., is an internal radiation therapy system to treat breast cancer following a lumpectomy.

· The MammoSite RTS is a device that is used to deliver interstitial brachytherapy.

· The MammoSite RTS is subject to physicians' clinical judgment in consultation with their patients.

· A catheter (a tube for insertion into a body passage or cavity) is temporarily implanted into the lumpectomy cavity.

· The catheter tip is surrounded by an approximately two-inch-diameter balloon that can be inflated with a mixture of saline (salt water) and contrast (for imaging purposes), to conform to the size of the lumpectomy cavity.

· The catheter can be implanted at the time of the lumpectomy or up to ten weeks after.

· The patient reports to the hospital or clinic for treatment on an outpatient basis where a radioactive "seed" is temporarily inserted within the inflated balloon, beginning a one to five day sequence of treatments.

· MammoSite RTS may be used in a course of about ten treatments over five days or as a boost to external beam radiation.

· No source of radiation remains in the patient's body between treatments or after the final procedure.

· When the therapy is concluded, the balloon is deflated and the MammoSite RTS catheter is easily removed.

Temporary implants are frequently used to irradiate the tumor bed from which a soft tissue sarcoma has been surgically removed. Marlene, a 45-year-old cosmetician, had a soft tissue sarcoma removed from the back of her right thigh. At the same time in the operating room, an interstitial implant of the tumor bed was performed.

An implant is performed by piercing the tissue at an appropriate angle with long, hollow needles. Hollow, flexible plastic catheters are inserted into the needles as those needles are removed. The catheters are fastened via metal tabs at their entry and exit sites. The metal tabs look like large clothing snaps. The sources of radioactive material are then introduced into the hollow catheters, and the metal tabs are crimped to secure the isotopes in place.

Temporary implants might remain in place for several days. Hospitalization is required because the patient is radioactive until the isotopes are removed. Radiation precautions must be taken by visitors and by nursing personnel to limit their exposure. This type of brachytherapy is called **low dose rate brachytherapy**.

Alternatively, **high dose rate brachytherapy** via an **afterloader** might be used. (High dose rate brachytherapy is temporary. High dose rate and low dose rate brachytherapy each have different advantages.)

The afterloader is a tungsten alloy shielded, portable machine, which contains a single radioactive source that remains attached at all times to the tip of a cable. (See Figure 8-2.) The cable is wrapped around an approximately three-inch-wide spool. (The opposite end of the cable remains attached to the spool at all times.) One or more approximately two-and-a half-foot transfer tubes are attached from the outside of the afterloader to the patient's implant or applicator via an approximately three-inch long, slender, metallic adapter.

Then, a computerized treatment control station directs the source from the afterloader into a patient's brachytherapy applicator or implant. The treatment control station positions the source and determines how long the source remains in any one position along the length of the applicator or implant. This way, the source is placed in multiple positions along the length of the applicator or implant. Such brachytherapy commonly avoids the need for hospitalization, bed rest, or radiation precautions because the radioactive material is removed after several minutes of treatment.

In high dose rate interstitial prostate implants, only the exit site of the catheter is accessible, as the entry site is deep within the prostate gland. In that scenario, a **template** (see Figure 8-3) is **sutured**, or stitched, to the skin. Several treatments are delivered over a 24- to 48-hour period, so this type of high dose rate brachytherapy implant is an inpatient procedure.

Most brachytherapy implants and insertions are performed in the sterile conditions of an operating room. **Local, spinal, epidural,** or **general anesthesia** is administered as needed. Some insertions, vaginal cylinder insertions for example, do not require anethesia, nor do they need to be performed in an operating room.

Restriction of activity can be anticipated with high dose rate prostate implants and with vaginal or uterine insertions. Bed rest is necessary to prevent displacement and dislodging of the applicator(s). For implants of the mouth, oral feedings are withheld until the implant is removed.

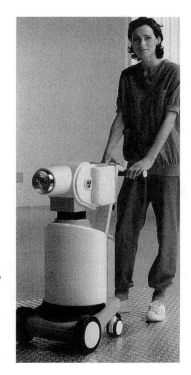

Fig. 8-2. The high dose rate remote afterloader is a portable apparatus that is used to deliver brachytherapy. (microSelectron-HDR, Nucletron Corp. Photo © 1995 by Nucletron Corp., Columbia, MD. All rights reserved. Used with permission.)

TANDEM AND OVOID INSERTION

Women with cervical cancer or endometrial (uterine) cancer, who have not undergone a hysterectomy, nearly always need brachytherapy, with or without external beam radiation therapy. The most common procedure is the intracavitary insertion of **tandem and ovoids**. These are smooth, metal applicators, with the tandem being thinner than a pencil. (See Figure 8-4.)

Kate (introduced in Chapter 2 in the section on brachytherapy) was diagnosed as having early stage cervical cancer. She was not a candidate for a hysterectomy because of significant heart disease. Kate, however, was eligible for curative treatment with a tandem and ovoids insertion.

The procedure was done in the operating room under sterile conditions and under anesthesia. Kate's gynecologist accompanied me during the procedure.

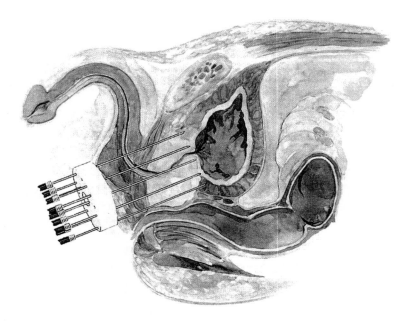

Fig. 8-3. High dose rate prostate implant. (Photo © 1995 by Nucletron Corporation. All rights reserved. Used with permission.)

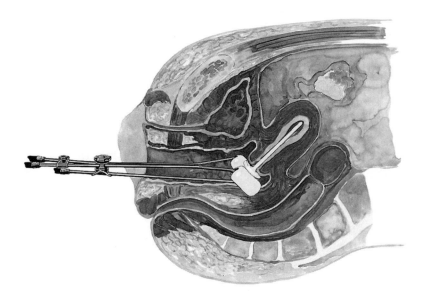

Fig. 8-4. A tandem and ovoids insertion. The tandem is inserted into the canal of the uterus. The ovoids are inserted along the sides of the tandem, where they are placed at the top of the right and left of the vagina. (Photo © 1995 by Nucletron Corporation. All rights reserved. Used with permission.)

Kate's legs were placed into stirrups to expose the vagina. Her vaginal area was cleaned with iodine solution. A catheter was inserted into her bladder to evacuate her urine into a bag. Then an instrument called a **weighted speculum** was inserted into the bottom of her vagina to retract the vagina's back wall. A **right angle speculum** was used to retract the front wall of the vagina. The top of Kate's cervix was grasped with an instrument called a **tenaculum**. This way, her cervix was clearly visualized. Four tiny metallic clips were injected into Kate's cervix so that the cervix might be identified on x-rays.

To prevent **perforation**, or puncturing of the uterus by the tandem, the depth of Kate's uterine canal was first determined with the use of an instrument called a **sound**. It is smooth and looks like a one-foot long straight metal wire that is much thinner than a pencil. The sound was gently inserted into Kate's cervix and uterus. When it was withdrawn, I was able

105

to measure the depth of her uterus. The length of the tandem was then adjusted by a stopper attached to the tandem.

After Kate's cervix was dilated a fraction of an inch with the dilators that are used for a D&C, the tandem was inserted into the cavity of her uterus. One ovoid was inserted on the right of the tandem into the right side of her vagina, and the other ovoid was inserted into the left side.

After the ovoids were introduced, the system was secured in place via gauze packing. The two **specula** were removed from Kate's vagina. A catheter was inserted into her rectum, and contrast material was instilled into the bladder catheter to enable visualization of these organs on x-rays. The rectal catheter was removed after the x-rays had been taken.

Kate was moved to the recovery room. While she was there, our physicist calculated the dose of radiation that her cervix, uterus, pelvic lymph nodes, bladder, and rectum would receive from the radioactive sources.

Patients who undergo low dose rate brachytherapy need to remain in bed between 48 and 72 hours. Medication that causes constipation is given to prevent patients from having a bowel movement. Patients are able to move their legs, but they aren't able to sit up, as they might dislodge the insertion.

The radioactive sources are loaded in the patient's hospital room. As I previously stated, visitors and health care workers must observe radiation precautions. When the insertion is removed, some patients require pain medication, as the vagina might feel irritated. The bladder catheter is removed as well.

Some patients require more than one insertion whether they are undergoing low or high dose rate brachytherapy. If so, the procedures are spaced approximately two weeks apart. Kate underwent four insertions, each spaced one to two weeks apart.

Several hours after Kate received each fraction of high dose rate brachytherapy, she went home. The actual radiation treatment took approximately 20 minutes. She was in the hospital a total of five hours each time.

Kate was told that once she went home, she had to avoid putting anything in her vagina for at least a week, because the dilated cervix was a conduit for infection. Once her cervix closed and her vaginal irritation subsided, Kate used vinegar and water vaginal douches and resumed intercourse.

VAGINAL CYLINDER INSERTION

A vaginal cylinder is used to treat the lining of the vagina in women who have undergone hysterectomy for cervical and endometrial cancer. Ruth (introduced a little earlier in this chapter) underwent the insertion of a vaginal cylinder. The procedure was performed in the operating room. Ruth's legs were placed in stirrups. The smooth, rounded cylinder was fully inserted into her vagina and secured in place with a single stitch through the bottom of her vagina. (See Figure 8-1.)

Ruth underwent high dose rate brachytherapy. Her brachytherapy session lasted 15 minutes and then she went home. She underwent two additional brachytherapy sessions spaced one week apart. At home, Ruth used vinegar and water douches as needed. She resumed intercourse once her vaginal irritation subsided.

PROSTATE SEED IMPLANTS

Jack (the 63-year-old art dealer whose condition was described in Chapter 2 in the section on brachytherapy) underwent a prostate seed implant eight weeks before his external beam radiation therapy for high-risk prostate cancer. Tony, a 71-year-old retired IRS agent with intermediate-risk prostate cancer, underwent external beam radiation therapy four weeks before having his seed implant performed.

Jack's and Tony's prostate seed implants were performed in two stages. First came the planning. Each patient had his legs placed into stirrups to expose the **perineum**, the area between the scrotum and the rectum. A **transrectal ultrasound probe** was inserted into the rectum. Attached to it is a square-shaped template, which rests against the perineum. (Figures 8-5 and 8-6 show pictures of such a template.) The template has a grid printed with letters horizontally and numbers vertically. This grid serves as a reference, providing the geometric conditions for establishing how the implant will be reproduced at the time of the actual seed implant.

Multiple ultrasound pictures of the prostate glands of each patient were taken. With computerized technology, the geometry of Tony's and Jack's prostates was reproduced on paper. The physicist then determined how many seeds needed to be introduced into the prostate for each man, and in what locations, in order to deliver the desired dose.

The prostate seed implants were performed in another setting — in the operating room under sterile conditions. Anesthesia was administered: Jack opted for general anesthesia and Tony chose spinal anesthesia. Once again, each man had his legs placed in stirrups, and sterile drapes were placed over his legs and abdomen. The penis and perineum were sterilized with iodine solution. A catheter was introduced into the penis and bladder to evacuate urine into a bag.

The transrectal ultrasound probe and template were then put back in place, using ultrasound guidance, to reproduce the spatial conditions that the prostate gland had assumed during planning. Radiation precautions were undertaken.

Following the plan, the seeds were inserted into the proper location within each man's prostate by piercing the skin of the perineum. The apparatus used resembles an elongated, narrow syringe. (See Figure 8-5 for a photo of the applicator.) This applicator contains a cartridge holder into which the cartridge containing the radioactive seeds is loaded. When the plunger of the applicator is withdrawn, a seed drops into the proper track. As the plunger is pressed forward, the seed is carried to the desired position.

As this procedure was carried out for Jack and for Tony, multiple areas of the perineum were pierced and rows of properly spaced seeds were implanted. The template and ultrasound probe were then removed. The implant procedure took 20 minutes to complete. X-rays of each man's pelvis were taken so the physicist could verify the dose distribution of the implant. (Figures 6-3 and 6-4 show a completed implant.)

It was necessary to keep the urinary catheter in each patient's bladder and penis for several days because the procedure causes **edema**, or swelling, of the prostate. Edema can cause **urinary retention**, the inability to void urine. To collect the urine while the catheter is in place, a bag was secured to the catheter tubing and to one leg of the patient. The catheter was safely removed within several days.

Other potential side effects, which each man was apprised of, include infection, bleeding, urinary frequency, urinary leakage, and impotence. Fortunately, most of the symptoms Tony and Jack experienced improved with the passage of time.

To protect others from radiation, each was told to refrain from hugging small children and women who might be pregnant, and not to hold

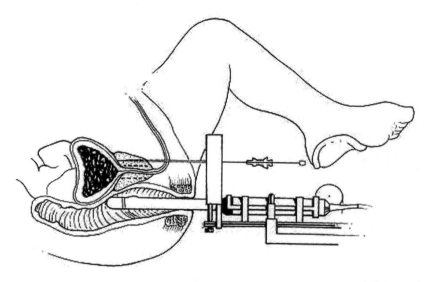

Fig. 8-5. Prostate Seed Implantation. (Drawing Courtesy of Peter Grimm, D.O., Executive Director, Seattle Prostate Institute.)

a child on his lap. These precautions needed to be observed for several weeks, until the **radiation safety officer** determined that each man's radioactivity had decayed to background level.

SYSTEMIC ISOTOPE THERAPY

Radioactive isotopes can be administered in pill form or via the intravenous route. Examples include radioactive iodine for the treatment of thyroid cancer, and Metastron (Nycomed-Amersham Products), which is radioactive strontium for the treatment of the bony metastases from prostate and breast cancer. Several other radioactive isotopes are also used as **unsealed internal radiation therapy**.

Hassan, an 82-year-old retired chemist, had diffuse and painful bone metastases secondary to prostate cancer. He was unable to tolerate the side effects of pain medication. Therefore, he received Metastron. After eight weeks his pain level had diminished substantially. His bone scan (an imaging study of the skeleton) was repeated, and many of Hassan's lesions had resolved.

109

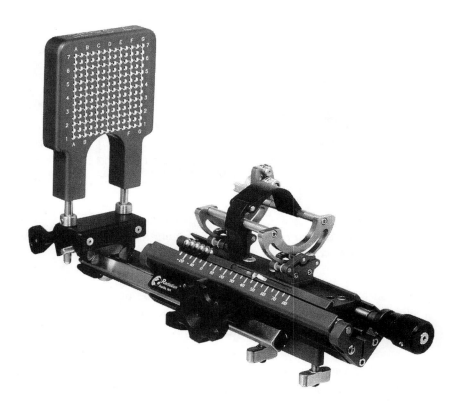

Fig. 8-6. Template for prostate seed implants. (Precision Prostate Stepper, MED-TEC, Inc. Photo © 2001 by MED-TEC, Inc. All rights reserved. Used with permission.)

STEREOTACTIC RADIOSURGERY

The term **radiosurgery** is a misnomer, as there is no cutting involved. Radiosurgery is actually a refined form of external beam radiation therapy. It can be administered with the linear accelerator, with proton beam therapy, or with a **gamma knife**.

Radiosurgery uses a large number of narrow, precisely aimed, highly focused beams of radiation. The beams are aimed at the target from multiple directions and they intersect at a specific point.

Radiosurgery is ideal for treating a very small, well-defined lesion. Radiosurgery can be delivered in multiple fractions or in a single, large dose.

Stereotactic radiosurgery was originally designed to treat benign and malignant brain lesions. Its use has been extended to treat other body sites. Radiosurgery can be delivered before conventional external beam radiation therapy, after conventional external beam radiation therapy, or as a sole radiation therapy modality.

Because the target is so small, the patient needs to be immobilized very well. Treating benign and malignant lesions of the head uses a stereotactic frame or immobilizer to limit motion and to reproduce the treatment position if more than one treatment will be delivered. (See Figure 8-7 for a photograph of the head frame.) For other body sites, alphacradles (Figures 5-7 through 5-9) and Vac-Lok Bags (Figure 5-10) are useful.

Nadia, a 22-year-old economics student, had a nonmalignant tumor, a meningioma, on the right side of her brain near the inner ear. She was experiencing intolerable ringing in her right ear and dizziness. She refused surgery and chose to be treated with stereotactic radiosurgery. Follow-up **MRI** scans demonstrated vast improvement of the tumor. Nadia's vertigo and ringing in her ear stopped.

TOTAL BODY IRRADIATION

Total body irradiation is intended to eradicate cancer cells throughout the entire body in patients who will be undergoing bone marrow and stem cell transplants. Total body irradiation causes enough suppression of the patient's immune system to prevent rejection of the donor marrow. When the recipient's body accepts the donor marrow, the process is called **engraftment**.

Another goal of total body irradiation is the eradication of genetically abnormal **clones** of cells (a group of identical cells that originated from a single cell) in disorders such as Fanconi's anemia.

Total body irradiation is usually done twice daily, with six hours between fractions and takes two weeks to complete. The procedure is performed with the patient standing up, lying down, or alternating between the two. Treatments are usually delivered from both the front and the back of the patient. Highly specialized shielding is used to protect the lungs and appropriate eye shields are used.

INTRAOPERATIVE RADIATION THERAPY

Intraoperative radiation therapy takes place in the operating room at the same time as surgery. A single, large dose of radiation therapy, usually via electron beam, is delivered to a tumor, which has been surgically exposed. The normal, surrounding organs are retracted away from the tumor. Sterile conditions are maintained. The actual radiation therapy takes place in a room that has adequate shielding for scattered radiation.

Alternatively, intraoperative radiation therapy can refer to the insertion of brachytherapy seeds or catheters into tumor tissues, a procedure that's also performed in the operating room.

HYPERTHERMIA

Using heat to treat cancer is generally done in conjunction with radiation therapy. Hyperthermia works on the premise that tumor regression is enhanced by high temperature.

Normal body temperature is 98.6 degrees Fahrenheit. Hyperthermia can raise the temperature in tumor tissue to between 105.8 and 113 degrees Fahrenheit or higher.

There are several methods of applying heat to the tumor without causing the patient a burn. One means entails the use of a microwave-heating device. A square applicator transmits heat to the tumor through a temperature-controlled water containing bolus. The bolus is placed on the surface of the tumor bearing area.

A method to heat deeper tumors involves implanting a plastic catheter into the tumor. A microwave-heating antenna is then fit snugly into the catheter or hot water can be irrigated through the catheter.

PHOTODYNAMIC THERAPY

Photodynamic therapy takes place after the intravenous injection of a material that works as a **photosensitizer**. Tumor cells retain the injected drug for several days and become sensitive to a special type of light. Normal tissue eliminates it within several hours.

Light of a particular wavelength is aimed at the tumor, usually via a flexible scope introduced into a body site. The light destroys the photosensitive tumor cells.

The efficacy of this treatment depends upon the penetration of light into tissue. Photodynamic therapy has proven most helpful in esophageal cancer and lung cancer.

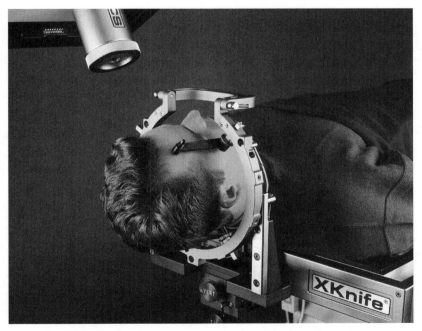

Fig. 8-7. Head frame for stereotactic radiosurgery. (HRA-IM Headframe, Radionics.™ Photo © 1998 courtesy of Radionics.™ All rights reserved. Used with permission.)

SPECIAL FORMS OF RADIATION THERAPY

RADIOIMMUNOTHERAPY

Radioimmunotherapy works on the principle of tagging a radioactive isotope to a **monoclonal antibody** that is highly specific for a tumor. A monoclonal antibody is a pure antibody, which is a protein. It is made in the laboratory by a single clone of cells. The radioactively tagged antibody is then attracted to the tumor as metal is attracted to a magnet, and it delivers therapy specifically to the tumor. This magic bullet selectively kills malignant cells while sparing normal tissue.

Monoclonal antibodies are used to treat leukemia, lymphoma, and several other malignancies. Monoclonal antibodies are administered via intravenous injection. Appropriate radiation precautions have to be implemented to limit radiation exposure to the public. Once the radioactivity has decayed to the background level, radiation precautions can be lifted.

CLINICAL TRIALS

Clinical trials, also known as protocols, are studies that take place on human subjects for the purpose of comparing different therapies (such as unproven treatments) to the existing standard therapy. A team of professionals, called an **Internal Review Board**, approves all clinical trials. The federal government carefully scrutinizes the board.

The advantage of clinical trials is that the new therapy being tested might turn out to be better than the existing standard. The patients who are eligible to participate in clinical trials are those who will not be harmed by receiving placebos. Therefore, patients participating in clinical trails are not merely being used as guinea pigs; they might be receiving better than the best-established care.

INTENSITY MODULATED RADIATION THERAPY (IMRT)

IMRT is a variation of 3-D conformal radiation therapy. Like 3-D conformal radiation therapy, IMRT conforms to the shape of the tumor. IMRT fields are treated with very small, multiple beams rather than with one uniform beam. Each different beam delivers a different dose to a different part of the tumor. The normal, surrounding tissue is protected from the high dose beams.

*"I learned very early in life that,
'without a song, the day would never end;
without a song, a man ain't got a friend;
without a song, the road would never bend —
without a song.'
So I keep singing a song."
– Elvis Presley*

CHAPTER 9

LIFE AFTER RADIATION THERAPY

Once you complete radiation therapy, you might experience a sense of relief. However, some patients have a sense of loss. While patients are coming for radiation therapy, they tend to feel as though things are under control. Once treatment is completed, some patients feel as though control has been lost.

This phenomenon is most commonly reported in patients who have undergone chemotherapy for breast cancer followed by radiation therapy and who have had a journey that lasted for nearly a year from the time of their breast cancer diagnosis. The sense of loss is a normal emotion, and reassurance is usually what such patients need.

Julia, a 47-year-old high school English teacher who had breast cancer, could not wait to put all of her treatments behind her. Once she reached her goal, however, she felt a sense of loss. The support that we gave to Julia expedited her road to emotional recovery.

After you complete your own treatments, you will be followed by your referring physician(s) and by your radiation oncologist. Such visits are called **follow-up examinations**. At a follow-up exam, your radiation oncologist will ask you questions and examine you. Any necessary blood tests and imaging studies (such as x-rays, CAT scans, MRI scans, and ultrasounds) will be ordered.

It is my policy to follow the guidelines issued by a panel of experts who form the National Comprehensive Cancer Network. However, I cannot stress how important it is for every radiation oncologist to use clinical judgment and not rely solely on printed guidelines. Therefore, tests might be ordered more often than the guidelines recommend, or less often; and different kinds of tests might be ordered in addition to the recommended panel. If your radiation oncologist has ordered any lab tests, you can anticipate your radiation oncologist's notifying you of your results in a timely fashion.

The frequency of follow-up visits also follows the guidelines, but variation might be necessary, again depending upon your individual needs. The duration of each radiation oncology follow-up visit varies; usually it lasts no more than 20 minutes.

Because many patients are followed by several physicians other than the radiation oncologist, I see them less frequently than recommended by the guidelines. My philosophy is that as long as one other qualified physician is performing the recommended follow-up examinations and studies, there is no necessity for patients to see their radiation oncologist as frequently.

Some patients find that coming for follow-up examinations causes them anxiety. I cannot emphasize strongly enough that it is important to treat the patient — not just the disease. As long as another competent physician is following the patient, I have no problem discharging that patient from radiation oncology follow-up. The radiation oncologist can always be re-consulted if needed.

It's my policy to request that any lab tests be forwarded to my office so they might be reviewed. In this way, even though I may not be seeing the patient, I am still following the patient's progress.

This policy was perfect for Peter, a 39-year-old stockbroker with testicular cancer. He was relieved that he would be able to see his urologist for follow-up examinations and did not need to return to the radiation oncology facility for this purpose.

On the other hand, some patients need the peace of mind of seeing their physicians often. Such patients will see their radiation oncologist more frequently than recommended "by the book." This was the case for Barbara, a 48-year-old bank teller, who completed — uneventfully — a course of radiation therapy for larynx cancer. She needed constant reassurance that not every twinge she felt was cancer-related.

116

Patients who receive radiation therapy should be followed throughout their lifetimes for three things:

- evidence of recurrent disease,
- identification and management of complications from radiation therapy, and
- surveillance for second malignancies.

Fortunately, the majority of patients experience no serious late effects from radiation therapy. Again, if the radiation oncologist is not performing such follow-up, another qualified physician can do so.

In my practice, I see most patients for their first follow-up examination six weeks after they complete radiation therapy, unless they have a problem that requires my seeing them sooner. I find that this timeframe is adequate for acute reactions to be resolved by time alone and for patients to adjust to any modifications they need in their lifestyles.

Anytime you are concerned, let your radiation oncologist know. Usually a means is available to reassure you. Also, remind yourself that you are *living* with cancer, not dying from cancer. Mindset is very important.

Claire, a most energetic and intelligent 43-year-old board of education administrator who was treated for breast cancer, learned to "find her song — and sing it." She made a point of going away with her husband during every school vacation period. Claire learned how to live after she became a breast cancer survivor.

Whatever your song is, be it music, art, gardening, cooking, traveling, woodworking, crafting, partying, theater, movies, TV, nature, sports, or working at your occupation, find your song — and sing it.

*"Never confuse a single defeat
with a final defeat."*
– F. Scott Fitzgerald

CHAPTER 10

FREQUENTLY ASKED QUESTIONS

Throughout the years that I have been practicing, I have been hearing these questions:

1. Will I be radioactive?

The way external beam radiation therapy is delivered can be compared to a light bulb. The radiation beam is either on or off. While you are receiving external beam radiation therapy, there is radioactivity in the room. Once the beam shuts off, there is no further radioactivity.

If you undergo brachytherapy, however, and if your sources of radiation are permanent, you are radioactive until your implanted radioactive sources decay to background level. If you have a temporary implant or insertion, you are radioactive until the sources are removed.

2. Will you put a lead shield on me?

No. A lead shield used during external beam radiation therapy is useless in **attenuating** — or reducing the potency of — the high-energy radiation therapy beam. Often, lead blocks are placed on the collimator of the radiation therapy machine to shape the field. Unblocked fields are collimated, or narrowed, to conform to the treatment field and to minimize unnecessary radiation exposure.

3. May I go in the sun?

I do not recommend sunbathing for anybody, because of the risk of skin cancer. However, sun exposure is inevitable when anyone walks outdoors. I recommend using sun block with at least SPF 30 on sun-exposed surfaces. If your irradiated area can be covered by wearing opaque, protective clothing, it is prudent to do so, because a sunburn on irradiated skin can complicate matters.

Going to the beach is pleasurable, so I would not discourage patients from doing so. However, it is wise to stay under an umbrella and wear as much protective clothing as possible in addition to sun block.

4. May I go swimming?

Yes. If you go swimming during a course of radiation therapy, be sure that when you come out of the water and dry yourself you apply moisturizer to the irradiated skin. If you experience ulceration of the irradiated skin, do not swim until the skin heals.

5. May I dye my hair?

Yes. As long as your head and neck area is not receiving radiation therapy, you may dye your hair. Be careful to avoid chemical hair-dye-induced burns of the skin on your neck and scalp.

6. What do the beam (port) films show?

Weekly beam films or port films are taken as a quality assurance measure to confirm that we are continuing to irradiate the proper area. The films show us if we are on target. These films are not diagnostic in purpose. Thus, we cannot tell from the films whether your tumor is regressing, growing, or remaining stable.

7. Will you do x-rays during the treatment?

Unless you have a specific symptom that warrants an x-ray, imaging studies are generally not ordered. Your radiation oncologist usually orders studies only if the findings might change what he or she would otherwise do.

8. What happens if I miss a treatment?

It's ideal to go through your treatment course without missing any days. In reality, however, people often do miss a day because of a holiday, vacation, inclement weather, illness, or machinery malfunction. As long as the treatment break is not prolonged, there is no consequence from missing a treatment. You do not need to start all over again; you simply continue where you left off.

9. Is there any special diet that I should follow? What about exercise?

During the course of radiation therapy, you can continue your normal diet. If you report any symptoms that warrant making modifications in your diet, your radiation oncologist will let you know. If your appetite is poor, the best thing is to eat many small portions frequently rather than three main meals a day. There is no restriction on eating before a radiation treatment.

If range of motion exercises are prescribed during and after radiation therapy, be sure to follow through. Otherwise, if you currently follow an exercise program, you may continue to do so as long as you feel well enough. There is no need to begin a strenuous exercise program during radiation therapy. Relaxation exercises, like those used in yoga and tai chi, are an excellent choice during and after radiation therapy. If you are overweight, you can begin a diet and exercise program after you have completed radiation therapy.

10. Can I continue using my medications?

Virtually no medications are contraindicated during the course of radiation therapy. You may therefore continue your prescribed medications. If you are taking any vitamins, your radiation oncologist might advise you to refrain from using antioxidant vitamins during the course of radiation therapy. (To understand the rationale, review the process of oxidation and free radical formation described in Chapter 2 in the section that explains how radiation therapy works.) Although no data exists to prove that antioxidants inhibit or interfere with radiation therapy, the theoretical possibility exists. Therefore, it is prudent to err on the side of caution and to hold off on antioxidants during the course of radiation therapy. You may resume their use as soon as you are done with radiation therapy.

11. Will I get sick?

Radiation therapy affects only the body sites being treated. If your stomach and intestinal area are not in the treatment field, you will not experience any nausea, vomiting, or diarrhea from radiation therapy.

12. Will I get burned?

Most tumors are treated with high-energy radiation therapy beams, which spare the skin. When more superficial beams are used for radiation treatment that's intended to treat the skin or the tissue just under the skin, a burn might occur. (Please see the discussion of burns and their management in Chapter 7.)

13. Will I lose my hair?

(Please see the discussion in Chapter 7 on radiation therapy to the head.)

14. When will I stop feeling so tired?

Fatigue during the course of radiation therapy is nonspecific. If fatigue is caused solely by radiation therapy, it should resolve within six months after you complete radiation therapy.

However, multiple factors can compound radiation therapy-induced fatigue. These include travel to receive radiation treatments, sleep deprivation, emotional distress, chemotherapy, medications, fluid and mineral imbalances, nutrition problems, anemia, hypothyroidism, diminished production of cortisol (a hormone produced in the body that gives people a sense of well-being), and miscellaneous factors. The mechanisms of radiation therapy-induced fatigue and cancer-related fatigue are not clear.

Treatment of fatigue is directed to the cause. If sleep deprivation is the cause for your fatigue, it's important to establish the reason for it. Is it because worry is interfering with your sleep? Is it because you are waking frequently to urinate? Are you having hot flashes secondary to hormonal therapy? Or are you experiencing pain that keeps you from sleeping? Once the source of your insomnia is determined, appropriate measures can be taken.

If you feel fatigued, you need not push yourself to do unnecessary activities. Exercise actually improves fatigue, but be sure to discuss physical exercise with your physician before you embark on a program. Yoga and tai chi are almost always excellent choices.

Follow your body's cues and rest or nap as much as needed, as long as it doesn't interfere with nighttime sleep.

It is prudent to list your activities according to how important they are to you. Don't be reluctant to ask for help and to delegate tasks when you can.

Establishing a structured daily routine is helpful. It is also beneficial to keep the objects that you use often within easy reach.

Using stress reducing methods, such as participating in a support group, deep breathing, meditation, visual imagery, prayer, talking to others, reading, listening to music, drawing, and any other activities that are pleasureable to you, is wise.

15. When will my pain start to improve?

Radiation therapy can take days or weeks to control pain. Therefore, you need to continue to use pain medication until radiation therapy has achieved its desired effect.

16. Will I become addicted to my pain medication?

Patients who use narcotics for cancer pain are using pain medication legitimately. Although you might develop a physical tolerance — which means you might need higher doses to achieve the same degree of pain relief — you will not become chemically dependent upon or psychologically addicted to narcotics. Withdrawal symptoms can be avoided by gradually reducing the dose instead of abruptly discontinuing narcotics.

17. I have no side effects. Does this mean that radiation therapy is not working?

No. Complications are not necessary in order to benefit from radiation therapy. In fact, many patients experience no side effects during radiation therapy and still achieve the desired, beneficial effect.

18. What happens to the destroyed cancer cells?

Cancer cells that have been destroyed by radiation therapy are scavenged away by your body's immune system, similar to the way your body's immune system destroys foreign matter that enters your body when you get a scratch or a cut.

19. Will I need somebody to accompany me to my treatments?

As long as you feel well enough to come by yourself for treatments, you need not bring anybody else. Of course, if you wish to bring friends or family members for moral support, you are welcome to do so. Radiation therapy is generally not a debilitating treatment. You should feel no different after your daily treatment. Therefore, you will be able to do everything you ordinarily do.

20. Can I ever receive radiation therapy again?

Each body site has its own tolerance for radiation therapy. This means that an area can receive a certain dose of radiation therapy and no more. Any body site can be retreated if its tolerance has not already been reached. A different body site can almost always be treated in the future. More than one body site can be irradiated at the same time. For example, patients who have multiple myeloma tend to receive radiation therapy to multiple bony sites.

21. Is there anything I need to do or not do while I am receiving radiation therapy?

The irradiated skin should be protected from the sun and from irritants such as deodorant soaps, antiperspirants, and perfumes. Patients who are being irradiated to the breast, chest wall, or mantle field may use alum crystal deodorant, which is sold in health food stores. The underarm on the opposite side of the irradiated breast or chest wall is not vulnerable to radiation-induced skin reaction; therefore, regular deodorant may be used on the unaffected side. A gentle, unscented soap is recommended.

Men receiving radiation therapy to the head and neck area should shave with an electric razor only. Women receiving radiation treatments to the breast, chest wall, or mantle area should not use a razor blade for shaving their underarms. An electric razor is acceptable.

If an extremity is being irradiated, such as a leg, a razor should not be used to shave the leg. An electric razor is reasonable. The skin of the leg should be moisturized with aloe after shaving.

22. What can I do to help myself during and after radiation therapy?

Follow your body's cues. For example, if you feel tired, make it a point to get your rest. Report any and all symptoms to your radiation oncologist, who can give you advice that is appropriate for your specific situation. (In Chapter 4 in the section on life and death issues, I discuss many of the self-help measures that patients can take. Chapter 9 offers suggestions as well.)

Remind yourself that you did not choose to get cancer, so give yourself a break. Find the balance between allowing yourself the rest and relaxation you need to recover from illness and the motivation and positive, optimistic outlook that is so important to complete recovery. Remember the support available through various agencies and do not hesitate to ask for help when you need it.

AFTERWORD

In most of the 20th century, a diagnosis of cancer was considered terminal. In the 21st century, however, physicians and patients have a wealth of diagnostic and treatment procedures and many people live with, and live past, cancer.

I wish you strength through this process, hope based on knowledge ... and a song to sing as well.

– Carol L. Kornmehl, M.D., F.A.C.R.O.

RESOURCES

There is an abundance of websites about cancer care. It is necessary for you to be cautious when you go online, as there are many "miracle cures" and inaccurate statements on the Internet.

1. American Board of Medical Specialties (ABMS)
   847-491-9091 www.abms.org

   The American Board of Medical Specialties is the umbrella organization for the 24 approved medical specialty boards in the United States. Lists of medical specialty boards, to find out if a particular doctor is board certified, are available for your perusal. A certified doctor locator service is also available.

2. American Cancer Society
   1-800-ACS-2345 www.cancer.org

   This network provides extensive information regarding services and organizations involved in the battle against cancer. Educational and support forums are available.

3. American Society for Therapeutic Radiology and Oncology (ASTRO).
   1-800-962-7876 www.astro.org

   ASTRO is a professional organization of physicians and scientists who specialize in radiation therapy. The society promotes the highest standards in patient care and provides opportunities for educational and professional development. ASTRO is actively involved in scientific research. A list of ASTRO members appears on this web site.

4. Cancer Care
   1-800-813-HOPE (4673) www.cancercare.org

This resource provides practical advice for those who are undergoing treatment for cancer and their families. Toll free telephone counseling is included.

5. *Candlelighters Childhood Cancer Foundation*
www.candlelighters.org

This organization was founded in 1970 by concerned parents of children with cancer.

6. *Clinical Trials Cooperative Group-National Cancer Institute (NCI)*
1-800-4-CANCER (1-800-422-6237) www.cancer.gov

As part of the National Institutes of Health, The National Cancer Institute coordinates a comprehensive research program of cancer cause, prevention, detection, diagnosis, and treatment.

7. *HEALTHFINDER*
www.healthfinder.gov

This United States government sponsored website serves as an index of health related resources, including other websites, databases, and publications.

GLOSSARY

The following terms either appear in this book or are used by health care providers. To help clarify the language, the terminology is defined in the context of radiation therapy.

ablate — To eliminate cancer cells.

acute side effects — Short-term, temporary reactions to radiation treatment.

adjuvant therapy — Treatment that is given in addition to the **primary therapy** to enhance the effectiveness of the **primary therapy.**

afterloader — A portable, tungsten alloy shielded machine that contains a single radioactive source. It is used for **high dose rate brachytherapy.**

akimbo position — A treatment position wherein the patient places his or her hands on the hips.

align — To straighten the patient on the treatment or simulation table so he or she is lying in a straight plane.

alopecia — Hair loss.

alphacradle — A custom-fitted device that immobilizes the patient and allows the daily treatment position to be reproduced.

anesthesia — The prevention of pain. **General anesthesia** puts the patient to sleep. **Local anesthesia** numbs a specific body part. **Regional anesthesia**, such as **spinal anesthesia** and **epidural anesthesia**, numbs the nerves that conduct sensation to a circumscribed body area.

antiemetic — A medication that prevents or relieves nausea and vomiting.

aquaplast mask — A custom-fitted device that fits over the patient's head and face to immobilize the patient and reproduce the position for daily treatment.

GLOSSARY

aquaplast strip — A custom-fitted treatment device that molds around the body part against which it is contoured, thereby allowing for reproduction of the patient's daily treatment position and immobilization of the patient.

attenuating — Reducing the energy of a radiation beam.

barium — A chalky-tasting pink or white liquid oral contrast or a chalky, white rectal contrast.

beam films — X-ray films of the treatment area(s) taken with the linear accelerator for comparison with simulation films; these enable the radiation oncologist to be certain that the radiation beam is hitting the correct target. They are also called **port films**.

belly board — A treatment device on which a patient lies face down; it has a rectangular hole for the belly to fall into, thereby reducing the volume of small intestine that remains in the treatment field(s).

benign — Not cancerous.

biologic therapy — Treatment that boosts the immune system's ability to fight cancer, also known as **immunotherapy**.

bite block — A device that is inserted into the patient's mouth to separate the upper and lower jaws; healthy tissue is thus moved out of the head and neck radiation field(s).

block cutter — An apparatus used to prepare the customized lead blocks that are used to protect the normal tissue that would otherwise be in the field during radiation treatment.

bolus — Rubbery material that is placed over the skin in the treatment **field** during radiation therapy. The x-rays and electron beam of the **linear accelerator** build up to their maximal dose a fraction of an inch below the skin surface. Bolus material acts as an artificial skin, enabling the radiation beam dose to build up to its maximum just underneath. The skin then receives the full dose of radiation instead of being spared from some of the dose.

boost — An extra radiation therapy dose delivered to the specific area that has the highest risk of harboring cancer cells. Also referred to as a **cone down**.

brachial plexopathy — Injury to the cluster of nerves at the lower neck that controls sensation and movement of the arm.

brachytherapy — Radiation therapy that is delivered from a short distance, such as directly on the skin surface, directly inside a body cavity, or directly within malignant tissues. A prostate seed implant is an example of the latter.

breast board — A rigid, slanted device meant for lying on from the waist up. It has an armrest to support the arm that is kept up and over the head during breast and chest wall radiation therapy.

cancer — A disease caused by abnormal cells that divide without control. These cells can spread into nearby tissues, spread to **lymph nodes**, and/or **metastasize** to other parts of the body.

cancer staging — Assessing the extent of the **primary tumor** and for the spread of cancer to the draining lymph nodes or distant body sites.

CAT scan — A computerized x-ray that obtains detailed images of the internal structures of a body site.

catheter — A flexible, hollow tube that can be introduced into the body.

centigray — A unit of radiation, equal to one 1-hundredth of a gray.

chemotherapy — Chemical substances or drugs given to combat cancer. Chemotherapy is delivered in the form of pills and intravenous injections.

chronic side effects — Side effects from radiation therapy of long duration that occur months or years after radiation therapy has been completed.

clamshell shield — A shield that is placed around a testicle to protect it from radiation exposure.

clinical neuropsychologist — A professional who is trained to assess and rehabilitate individuals with impaired mental acuity.

clone — A group of identical cells that originated from a single cell.

cobalt machine — A machine that derives radiation from a radioactive cobalt source of material and delivers external beam radiation therapy to treat cancer.

cognitive retraining — Rehabilitation of patients who have a significant impairment of their mental acuity.

collimator — The component of a linear accelerator that confines the radiation beam to a specific area.

cone down — An extra radiation therapy dose that is delivered to the specific area that has the highest risk of harboring cancer cells. Also known as a **boost**.

couch — The table of the **linear accelerator** and **simulator** on which the patient lies for treatment.

cranial prosthesis — A wig.

craniospinal axis — The body area relating to the brain and spinal cord.

cystourethrogram — An x-ray image of the bladder and the urethra (the tube that evacuates urine from the bladder to the outside of the body).

3-D conformal radiation therapy — Radiation beams that conform to the shape of a tumor and spare the healthy surrounding tissue. The tumor is outlined on a CAT scan; using a 3-D treatment planning computer, a customized treatment plan is developed.

definitive therapy — Any treatment used as the only therapy.

dilation — A procedure that stretches the narrowed **lumen** back to an appropriate diameter.

dilator — A device that is used to stretch a body cavity.

dosimetrist — A member of the radiation therapy team who plans and calculates the proper radiation therapy dosage.

dual energy linear accelerator — A linear accelerator that has two different high energies of x-rays. One energy is higher and the other is lower.

edema — Swelling of any body part.

electron beam — Radiation therapy that is delivered via a stream of negatively charged atomic particles.

endocrinologist — A physician who specializes in diagnosing and correcting hormonal aberrations.

engraftment — The acceptance (as opposed to the rejection) of a donor's bone marrow by the recipient's body.

epidural anesthesia — See **anesthesia**. A local anesthetic is instilled into the space between the soft tissue that lines the spine and the **vertebral body**.

erectile dysfunction — The inability to achieve or sustain an erection.

esophageal stricture — A significant narrowing of the esophagus, the tube that connects the mouth to the stomach.

external beam radiation therapy — Radiation treatment that is delivered by a machine, such as a **linear accelerator,** to the outside of the body to attack cancer cells.

field — The body area at which the radiation beam is directed. Also referred to as a **portal**.

fine motor skills — Tasks that are accomplished with the use of the arms, hands, and fingers, such as tying a shoelace, typing, using a computer mouse, and inserting a key into a lock.

fluoride — A chemical that prevents tooth decay.

fluoride gel carrier trays — Plastic-like devices that are contoured to the patient's upper and lower teeth , which the patient fills each day with fluoride gel, then wears on the teeth for several minutes daily. This measure reduces tooth decay.

fluoroscope — The instrument that is used for fluoroscopy.

fluoroscopy — Observing the internal body structures by means of x-rays.

follow-up examinations — Checkups that take place after radiation therapy has been completed.

fraction — Each individual, daily radiation treatment in a prescribed series of treatments.

free radicals — Highly reactive chemical species produced during radiation therapy.

gamma knife — A device that is used to deliver **radiosurgery** to treat brain lesions. High energy rays are derived from cobalt, and radiation beams are delivered at many different angles.

gamma rays — High energy waves emitted by radioactive substances.

general anesthesia — See **anesthesia.**

Gleason grade — The differentiation (how closely a tumor resembles normal tissue when thin slices of cancer tissue are studied under a microscope) of prostate cancer.

grays — See **centigrays.**

headrest — A special pillow that is used to support the head and neck during radiation therapy.

high dose rate brachytherapy — Internal radiation therapy that is delivered within minutes via a computer-driven machine, which controls the insertion and withdrawal of its radioactive source.

hospice — A facility or program designed to provide for the physical and emotional needs of terminally ill patients.

hyperextended — A patient position in which the neck is tilted back as far as it can go.

hyperfractionation — The administration of more than one radiation treatment in a day.

hypothyroidism — Diminished production of thyroid hormone by the thyroid gland.

immobilization device — A device used during simulation and treatment to keep a patient from moving and to reproduce the same position for daily treatments.

immunotherapy — See **biologic therapy**.

implant — See **interstitial brachytherapy**.

insertion — See **intracavitary insertion**.

intensity modulated radiation therapy (IMRT) — A variation of **3-D conformal radiation therapy**; IMRT conforms to the shape of the tumor. **Fields** are treated with multiple, very small beams rather with one uniform beam. Each beam delivers a different dose to a different part of the tumor. The normal surrounding tissue is protected from the high dose beams.

Internal Review Board — A panel of experts that approves clinical trials and is carefully scrutinized by the federal government.

internal radiation therapy — See **brachytherapy.**

internal scatter — The dissemination of radiation from within the body to non-exposed areas.

interstitial brachytherapy — Internal radiation therapy (brachytherapy) that is performed by the implantation of radioactive material into body tissues. It may be temporary or permanent.

intracavitary insertion — Internal radiation therapy (brachytherapy) that is performed via the insertion of radioactive material into a body cavity, such as the uterus and cervix.

intraluminal insertion — Internal radiation therapy (brachytherapy) that is performed via the insertion of radioactive material into a hollow body structure such as the esophagus and the lung (airway).

intraoperative radiation therapy (IORT) — A high dose of radiation therapy that is delivered to a tumor or tumor bed in the operating room.

ionization — The formation of negatively and positively charged particles.

irradiate — To treat with radiation.

isotopes — Radiation sources that have an unstable nuclear (center of the atom) composition.

laser beam — A thin beam of red light that is used to **align** patients during **simulation** and treatment.

lesion — **Benign** or **malignant** abnormal **tissue**.

L'Hermitte's sign — An electric shock sensation in the spine and tingling or pain in the hands that is produced by bending the head forward following radiation therapy to the upper spinal cord.

linear accelerator — A radiation therapy machine that uses electricity to create high-energy x-ray beams to treat disease.

local anesthesia — See **anesthesia**.

local control — Control of cancer at a particular body site, such as that of origin.

local treatment — A therapy that makes its impact on the immediate area to which it is applied. Examples are radiation therapy and surgery.

low dose rate brachytherapy — Internal radiation therapy that takes hours or days to complete.

lumen — The cavity of a hollow organ, such as the esophagus.

lumpectomy — The surgical removal of a breast tumor with a limited amount of normal, surrounding breast **tissue**.

lung board — A radiation therapy device that is useful when a patient must lie with his or her arms up over the head. It has handles that the patient grasps comfortably, thus facilitating the reproduction of the patient's daily treatment position.

lymph nodes — Pea-sized glands situated throughout the body that filter lymph, which is a clear fluid the body collects from its tissues. Cancer cells and infectious agents are among the entities collected in lymph nodes.

lymphedema — Swelling of a body part because of disruption of the flow of lymph, a clear fluid the body collects from its tissues.

MammoSite — A **catheter** that is implanted into the **lumpectomy** cavity of a breast so that **brachytherapy** might be administered to the **tumor bed**.

mantle — A classic radiation therapy field that encompasses lymph nodes of the neck, chest, and underarms that is often used to treat Hodgkin's disease.

margins — The borders of a surgically removed tumor.

medical oncologist — A physician who is specially trained at prescribing chemotherapy and hormonal therapy to treat cancer.

metastasis — A tumor that results from cancer cells that dislodged from the original tumor and spread to other parts of the body.

metastasize — Cancer cells that have dislodged from the primary tumor and have traveled, or spread, to distant body sites.

microscopic disease — A disease that can be detected only with a microscope, not on x-rays or by physical examination.

monoclonal antibody — A pure antibody (which is a protein) made in the laboratory by a single **clone** of cells (a group of identical cells that originated from a single parent cell). These antibodies have a specific affinity for cancer cells.

MRI Scan — A study that uses a magnet rather than x-rays to form images of the inside of the body.

multimodality therapy — The use of more than one type of therapy (**radiation** therapy, surgery, **chemotherapy**) to treat cancer.

multileaf collimator — A computer-driven blocking device of the linear accelerator that shapes the radiation beam.

neo-adjuvant radiation therapy — Radiation therapy that is delivered prior to surgery in an attempt to shrink a tumor and make it amenable to surgical removal.

neutral position — A radiation therapy position wherein the patient's neck is straight, instead of bent forward or backward.

neutron beam — A stream of uncharged atomic particles that can be generated by special radiation equipment.

nodule — A small tumor.

occupational therapist — A health care professional who is trained at rehabilitating patients in **fine motor** tasks, such as buttoning a shirt and tying a shoelace.

oncogenes — Genes that are responsible for hereditary cancers.

oncologist — A physician who is specially trained at treating patients with cancer.

ovoids — See **tandem and ovoids**.

oxidation — Decreasing the negative charge of an atom or ion (a charged particle) during radiation therapy.

palliation — Treatment that is not curative but that relieves symptoms from cancer, such as pain, bleeding, and obstruction.

pathology report — A report issued by a pathologist (a physician who studies diseases) after a surgical specimen or biopsy is examined.

perforation — Puncturing a hollow organ.

perineum — The area lying between the vagina and anus in females and between the scrotum and anus in males.

PET scan — An imaging study that helps to distinguish cancer from **benign tissue** and assesses the response of cancer to therapy. A patient is injected with a tiny amount of a radioactive material that is combined with a sugar. The test works on the principle that tumors metabolize (use up) more sugar than normal tissue.

photosensitizer — An agent that enhances a tumor's sensitivity to light.

physical therapist — A health care professional who is trained at rehabilitating patients via exercise and massage.

platelets — The component of blood that controls bleeding and clotting.

portal — The body area that is treated with radiation. Also referred to as a **field**.

port films — See **beam films**.

post-operative radiation therapy — Radiation therapy that is delivered after an operation has been performed.

pre-operative radiation therapy — Radiation therapy that is delivered before a planned operation.

primary therapy — Any treatment used as the only therapy.

primary tumor — The original cancer that can spread and give rise to **metastatic** tumors.

prophylactic surgery — Surgery to remove one or more organs (such as the breasts and ovaries) that are at a significant risk for the future development of cancer.

prosthesis — An artificial body part replacement.

proton beam — A specialized form of radiation therapy that generates a stream of positively charged subatomic particles. It is useful for treating specific tumor types, such as pituitary tumors.

PSA level — A blood test that measures Prostate Specific Antigen, a chemical made by the prostate gland.

rad — A unit of radiation, equal to one centigray. See **centigray**.

radiation — Waves or streams of particles that carry energy.

radiation-induced lung fibrosis — Scar tissue built up in the section of lung tissue that has been exposed to radiation therapy. This represents a chronic side effect.

radiation nurse — A nurse who is a member of the radiation treatment team, coordinates a patient's care, and manages side effects from radiation therapy.

radiation oncologist — A physician who has been specially trained at treating diseases with **radiation therapy**.

radiation physicist — A member of the radiation therapy team who oversees the radiation machinery and its delivery of the correct amount of radiation to the treatment site(s).

radiation pneumonitis — A form of pneumonia induced by radiation therapy; it represents a short-term complication from radiation therapy.

radiation safety officer — A physicist who oversees the radioactive material that is used to treat a patient internally so it poses no public health risk once the patient is released from the hospital.

radiation therapist — A member of the radiation treatment team who positions the patient on the **simulator** and **linear accelerator** tables and who runs the equipment for **simulation** and treatment.

radiation therapy — The treatment of diseases via penetrating beams of high energy waves or streams of particles.

radiation treatment — See **radiation therapy.**

radioactive — A substance that emits high energy rays or particles.

radiologist — A physician who specializes in interpreting imaging studies and who performs invasive procedures under x-ray guidance.

radiosensitizer — A medication that enhances a patient's response to radiation therapy.

radiosurgery — A radiation therapy technique that uses a large number of narrow, precisely aimed, highly focused beams of radiation. The beams are aimed from many directions and intersect at a specific point.

radiotherapy — See **radiation therapy**.

radiotherapy technologist — See **radiation therapist.**

range of motion exercises — Exercises that are performed by a patient to maintain the span of movement of a joint.

reconstructive surgery — An operation that is performed to minimize the cosmetic and functional impairment from cancer surgery.

recurrence — The relapse of cancer, either in the original site, lymph nodes, or a distant site, after a cancer-free interval.

red blood cells — The component of blood that delivers oxygen to body tissues.

regional anesthesia — See **anesthesia**.

remote brachytherapy — See **high dose rate brachytherapy**.

right angle speculum — A gynecologic instrument used to retract the top of the vagina so that the canal of the vagina and the cervix can be examined.

scout film — An x-ray film that is taken of a specific area before the patient ingests or is injected with contrast material.

seeds — Tiny, slender radioactive metal pellets that are implanted into the prostate gland to deliver **brachytherapy** for prostate cancer.

simulation — A mapping-out session in which the treatment area is defined and marked on the patient and/or any of the patient's immobilization devices.

simulator — The piece of equipment on which simulation is accomplished.

Sitz bath — A shallow pan that fits on the toilet bowl; it is filled with warm water. It is soothing to the skin of the **perineum** when a patient sits on it.

sound — An instrument that is used to measure the depth of the uterus. A sound is smooth, approximately one foot in length, and is much thinner than a pencil.

spatial cooperation — The concept that hormonal therapy can eliminate metastatic prostate cancer cells that will not be encompassed by the radiation treatment **portals** of the prostate gland.

speculum — A smooth instrument that is used to retract tissue to aid in seeing an organ. An example is a speculum that is inserted into the vagina to enable examination of the cervix.

speech pathologist — A health care professional who specializes in the diagnosis and treatment of disorders of speech and language.

spinal anesthesia — See **anesthesia**. A local anesthetic solution is injected into the fluid that bathes the spinal cord.

spinal cord compression — Pressure put upon the spinal cord by a tumor or bony fragment of the spine. If untreated, it can result in permanent paralysis and/or disturbance of bowel and bladder function. **Spinal cord compression** is one of the indications for emergency radiation therapy.

stereotactic — Directing a radiation beam in three dimensions to reach a specific, localized area of the body.

stereotactic radiosurgery — See **radiosurgery.**

subtotal brain irradiation — Radiation therapy of less than the whole brain.

superior vena cava syndrome — Compression of the major vein of the chest (the superior vena cava) by a tumor mass that results in an increase of veins on the chest wall and the swelling of the face, neck, and arm(s).

surgical clips — Metallic bits that resemble staples or pellets. Surgeons place clips around a tumor or **tumor bed.** Because the clips are evident on x-rays, the radiation oncologist can customize the shape(s) of the radiation beam(s).

surgical oncologist — A physician who performs operations to remove cancer.

suture — A stitch.

synergism — Interaction of radiation and drugs such as chemotherapy agents, which produces a greater total effect than the sum of the individual effects.

systemic therapy — Therapy distributed via the bloodstream to the entire body.

tandem and ovoids — An apparatus that is used to insert brachytherapy sources for gynecologic cancers, such as endometrial cancer or cervical cancer. The tandem is a narrow, smooth tube that is introduced into the uterus; ovoids are a pair of smooth tubes that fit along the sides of the tandem. One ovoid is inserted into the right side of the vagina and the other into the left.

tattoos — Permanent marks that are made on the skin to aid in daily treatment set-up.

technologist — See **radiation therapist.**

telangiectasis — A spidery, thin blood vessel that is visible on the skin. (Plural: telangiectases.)

teletherapy — Radiation therapy from a relatively far distance of about 1-2 feet, such as that delivered by a linear accelerator.

template — A grid of horizontal letters and vertical numbers that is etched into a rectangular plate. This device is used during prostate seed implants to determine where to place each seed.

temporomandibular joint (TMJ) — The hinge joint of the jaw bones.

tenaculum — An instrument used to grasp the uterine cervix.

therapist — See radiation therapist.

tissue — A group of similar cells and the substance between them.

tolerance — The amount of radiation an organ or body site can receive without becoming damaged.

total skin electron beam — Irradiation of the entire skin surface with an electron beam; traditionally used for patients who have mycosis fungoides, a lymphoma of the skin.

transrectal ultrasound probe — A smooth, rounded device inserted into the rectum to obtain ultrasound images of the prostate.

treatment port — The body area at which the radiation beam is directed. Also called a **field.**

tumor — A mass of either benign (non-cancer) cells or malignant (cancer) cells.

tumor bed — The **tissue** surrounding a tumor, which has been surgically removed.

ultrasound — The use of sound waves to generate images of internal body structures.

unsealed internal radiation therapy — A form of **brachytherapy** that entails the introduction of a radioactive material into the bloodstream or body cavity. An example is the administration of a radioactive iodine pill, which is absorbed into the bloodstream, to deactivate the function of the thyroid gland.

urethral stricture — A significant narrowing of the tube that evacuates urine from the bladder to outside the body.

urinary retention — The inability to evacuate urine.

Vac-Lok Bag — A device used for radiation therapy. It reproduces the patient's daily position and immobilizes the patient. The patient is positioned in the device and the air is suctioned out; Styrofoam pellets then fill in the air spaces and form a mold.

vaginal dilator — A rigid, plastic tampon-shaped device that a woman inserts into her vagina for several minutes to stretch the tissues and keep them pliable.

vaginal marker — A smooth, plastic device, shaped like a tampon. It is inserted into the vagina so it might be identified on x-rays.

vertebral bodies (vertebrae) — The bones that make up the spine.

weighted speculum — See **specula**. This type of speculum has a weight built into the handle that pulls the bottom of the vagina down, enabling the examination of the uterine cervix.

white blood cells — The component of blood that fights infection.

x-ray — Low-dose radiation used to take pictures of internal body structures (for example, a chest x-ray); also high-dose radiation used to treat disease (such as radiation therapy).

INDEX

-W-

weakness 34, 35, 94
weighted speculum 105, 144
weight gain 36
white blood count 74
wig 76, 134
worry 27, 34, 99, 122

-X-

x-ray 5, 6, 10, 15, 19, 45, 46, 47,
    50, 51, 53, 54, 55, 56, 57, 58,
    64, 65, 66, 67, 68, 69, 70, 90,
    93, 94, 105, 106, 108, 115,
    121, 132, 133, 134, 135, 137,
    138, 140, 141, 142, 143, 144

-Y-

yoga 28, 121, 122

About the Author

Carol L. Kornmehl, M.D., F.A.C.R.O., is a board-certified radiation oncologist. Dr. Kornmehl is a consultant on the medical staff of the following hospitals in New Jersey: The Medical Center of Ocean County, Kimball Medical Center, Our Lady of Lourdes Medical Center, Virtua Health, and Kessler Memorial Hospital.

Dr. Kornmehl is a graduate of the State University of New York at Downstate Medical Center, where she also completed her radiation oncology residency. She was Medical Director of New Jersey Radiation Therapy, Brick, New Jersey from 1998–2002 and Medical Director of Radiation Oncology at Monmouth Medical Center, Long Branch, New Jersey from 1994–1997.

Dr. Kornmehl is Clinical Assistant Professor of Radiation Oncology at Hahnemann University Hospital. Previously, she was Assistant Professor of Clinical Radiology at the University of Medicine and Dentistry of New Jersey.

Dr. Kornmehl has received multiple honors, including listing in Who's Who Among Rising Young Americans; How to Find the Best Doctors: New York Metro Area; National Registry of Who's Who; and America's Registry of Outstanding Professionals. She has been elected a Fellow of the American College of Radiation Oncology for her exemplary service to the field.

Professional memberships include: American Society for Therapeutic Radiology and Oncology, The Oncology Society of New Jersey, The American College of Radiology, The New Jersey Academy of Medicine, The Cancer Institute of New Jersey, The Eastern Cooperative Oncology Group, and The Radiologic Society of New Jersey.

As an author, Dr. Kornmehl has been published in scientific textbooks and journals. She may be reached through www.rtsupportdoc.com, her website.

**Do you know someone who could benefit
from a copy of this book?**

**Order from your local bookstore
or mail in the order form on the next page.**

Quantity	Title	Price	Total
	The Best News about Radiation Therapy: How to Cope and Survive	14.95	

SUBTOTAL.. $ _____

NJ residents add 6% sales tax .... _____

Shipping & Handling:..._____

* If your total order ranges between $ 14.95 – $ 49.99 US.....add 25%
* If your total order ranges between $ 50.00 and up..............add 15%

TOTAL $_____

This form is for orders within the United States only.
Money Order payable to
Academic Radiation Oncology Press
or credit card only:

AMEX   Discover   MasterCard   Visa

Card #_____ Expiration Date: _____

Signature:_____

Thank you for your order!

Name _____

Address _____

City_____ State _____ ZIP_____

Phone (_____)_____ E-mail _____
Mail to:
Academic Radiation Oncology Press
103 Candlewood Commons, Howell, NJ 07731
Or FAX to: (732) 364-6950